RAISE
YOUR
HDL

Healthy Deserve Level

For Successful Dental Teams

GARY KADI

First Edition January 2009
Second Edition May 2009

Published by Gary Kadi
www.garykadi.com

ISBN: 978-0-9820719-0-8

Printed in the United States of America

Book Design by Dotti Albertine

Gratitude

Thank you, Thank you, Thank you to my fellow High HDLers...

To our family of clients, who are always looking beyond success and are the source and inspiration for this book.

To my team, for your dedication, grace, and love in our mission to profoundly and measurably enhance the quality of people's lives.

To my dear family, whose unconditional love and support is very much appreciated.

To my wife Judith and my son Rome for the blessed life we have and your patience and support in allowing this project to happen.

To my 92-year-old grandmother Vera, whose spirit and wisdom have contributed to this work.

To my coaches, Alice and Julia, for your unwavering support and accountability.

To Michael Levin and his team for your brilliance in organizing and structuring this book.

Contents

*In practice and in life,
you do not get what you deserve.
You get what you THINK you deserve.
Nothing more. Nothing less.*

—GARY KADI

Welcome to the second edition of *Raise Your HDL!* I'm humbled by the rapid success we've achieved and honored that you are taking the time to enjoy this book.

Wherever I go, people ask me the same question: Why a book about the inner psychology of dentists and their team members? Why not another book about how to succeed financially with new tips and tricks for growing a practice?

I would like to answer that question by telling you a story.

There was a dentist who read my first book, *Million Dollar Dentistry*, and quickly embraced the principles it offers in order to build a thriving practice—a happy team; the doctor chair-side for a much higher percentage of his day than ever before; rockin' cash flow; patients accepting treatment and getting the care they need; and the entire team motivated, incentivized, and winning big-time.

After reading *Million Dollar Dentistry*, this dentist, whom we'll call Tom, called us in to work with him and his team. Tom's dream collection amount was $120,000 a month, which was slightly more than double what he'd been making prior to becoming acquainted with the ideas in *Million Dollar Dentistry*.

From our perspective, Tom was a dream client—he took the ideas we proposed and ran with them, reorganizing his entire practice along the lines we suggested. He gave his hygienists a full hour in order to do what they love to do—give patients the care they need and educate them on their unique problems and probable solutions of the soft and hard tissue conditions. Hygienists are born educators, and Tom's team finally felt empowered to help the patients recognize exactly what was going on in their mouths. This is, of course, the first step in getting patients to accept cases—the hygienist points out what's necessary using their intraoral cameras on EVERY visit. Then the doctor comes in and receives a Trust Transfer™ from the hygienist, allowing him to offer her/his agreement on the areas to be treated, which have been previously established in the practice's Healthy Mouth Baseline™.

From there, the patient is Trust Transferred to the treatment coordinator's office, which Tom set up, making use of a room that had been previously little more than a graveyard for old and outmoded computer equipment and stacks of files. There, the treatment coordinator sits down with the patient and works out the specifics of the treatment and essentially closes the case on the spot, also helping the patient choose from an array of payment options, including Care Credit and what we call a Pay Today courtesy. All this, and the other changes Tom enacted, meant that he was now free to do what he loved best: focus on practicing dentistry with his patients, giving them his expert care, and, not coincidentally, raising the morale in the office and also in his monthly collections.

Before long, Tom reached that seemingly impossible target of $120,000 a month in gross collections.

And that's when the trouble began.

Something inside Tom freaked when he was making all that money, because the actions he took from that point forward were the exact opposite of what we had proposed.

First, he fired his treatment coordinator, on the grounds that she wasn't contributing to the overall success of the office—she was just an expensive salary that he wanted to dump.

Then he cut the hygienists' consultations back to forty-five minutes, thinking that if he could make $120,000 with them seeing eight patients a day, then maybe he could make $150,000 if they were seeing twelve.

This strategy backfired, of course, because the hygienists felt rushed and no longer had the time to educate the patients about the dental work they believed was necessary.

Then, when he came into the hygienists' area, instead of agreeing with what he saw—even though he knew they were right 99 percent of the time—he would invalidate their suggestions in front of the patient, leaving the patients confused as to whom they should trust.

The new bonus structure we had created, Tom believed, was eating into his profits, so he quietly scrapped it. As a result, two key members of his front desk team quit, leaving the office in complete disarray.

Before long, Tom was actually worse off than he was when he first read *Million Dollar Dentistry*. He was back to carrying around his own paychecks that he couldn't cash. Patients had gone back to their old habits of refusing treatment, canceling appointments at the last minute, or simply failing to show up. The remaining staff was demoralized and the office was in crisis. Trust was lost.

What had happened to Tom?

Very simply, *Tom was experiencing success he didn't believe he deserved.*

He called us back in and we went over everything that had happened, both on his rise to the top and then on his subsequent collapse. He agreed that there was nothing wrong with the ideas that we had presented. But he also told us that he had crossed an invisible line in his psyche— he was now making more money than he could have ever imagined. And something inside him was saying he couldn't do that.

So he quickly set out to sabotage the very system that had created all his success.

Tom is not alone. We've installed the *Million Dollar Dentistry* approach in hundreds of dental offices across the United States, Canada, and Great Britain in over a decade. We offer a better-than-risk-free return on investment guarantee—we take what you've collected over the past twelve months, add the value of the program, and then promise to collect at least that amount or stay on until we do. We do not "come close," because every doctor who has followed our guidance has indeed experienced the same sort of uplift in income and team morale that Tom witnessed.

At the same time, a handful of the doctors with whom we have worked have bumped up against the same problem that Tom faced. And it had nothing to do with the economy, the decline in housing values leading people to cut back on "optional" items like dental care, or any other external factor.

It all came down to the beliefs that the doctors had about what they deserved from life.

All too often, we discovered, the doctors were building their newfound success not on a solid internal foundation—what I call a Healthy Deserve Level—but instead on quicksand. They were outstanding at their work—their dentistry was faultless. But their mentality reflected a low Deserve Level. No matter how effectively their offices were now running, no matter how empowered their team members were to provide outstanding care, close cases, and radically increase the cash flow in the office, many of these doctors were mired in a mindset that did not allow them to enjoy the fruits of the hard work they had performed which was transforming their practices.

If you think back to the old *Saturday Night Live* sketch, "Wayne's World," one of their great catch phrases was, "We're not worthy!" That was a joke, and it reflected the innocent admiration that those guys had for their rock star heroes. But when a doctor or team member thinks, "I am not worthy," it's no joke. It's an indication that disaster is a heartbeat away.

When doctors possess a low Deserve Level, they are all too often coming from a mentality that dooms them to failure no matter how hard they work. It's a mindset rooted in blame, self-justification, impatience, laziness, procrastination, self-importance, and above all, an inability to trust themselves. The overall term that summarizes this approach to life is "poverty thinking." Poverty thinking relies on a sense that there is never enough and there will never be enough, and even if there were, the doctor doesn't feel worthy of having good things in his or her life. Hence *they* are not enough.

There's nothing funny about a low Deserve Level. And doctors are not the only ones who can experience it. Take a look at the world around us. On Wall Street, you had bankers and traders believing that no matter how hard they worked, they weren't going to have enough money. And they had plenty! So they cheated and fudged. They took advantage of regulatory loopholes. They created Ponzi schemes, both legal and illegal. And they took the economy down.

We see the same thing in sports, where athletes have destroyed their own careers and reputations because they were too afraid to rely on their own natural gifts. Instead, they used steroids and other performance-enhancing drugs, tainting their own records and creating a legacy of mistrust and disappointment for their fans.

In other words, it's hardly an exaggeration to say that we live in a culture mired in poverty thinking, in blaming others and not taking responsibility for our choices...and above all, in our own negative thoughts that underlie our actions.

Fortunately, there is a solution. And the solution is the topic of this book. The solution is understanding what it takes to raise one's Deserve Level.

If we're coming from the past, from a mentality we developed long ago that tells us we are unworthy and not enough, we're doomed. That's because our past thoughts and actions create the present in which we find ourselves. We like to think that *Million Dollar Dentistry* is the gold standard for re-crafting a dental practice and taking it to the next level. But it doesn't matter how good a program is if the person in charge—the doctor—doesn't believe that he or she is worthy of having it all. If we're coming from the past, and our past is all about negativity, we are certainly not going to be in a position to create the kind of present we want for ourselves.

In *Raise Your HDL*, you'll learn how to draw a line in the sand and put the past behind you, once and for all. You'll learn how to take the negative thinking that may have literally crippled your ability to enjoy life and maximize the income, joy, and love you experience instead. In this book, I'll show you how to create a future for yourself where your dental practice, your home life, and your overall lifestyle reflect the high level of success you deserve. I'll show you how to develop a mindset rooted in responsibility to yourself and others, contribution and generosity to the world around you, and freedom from fear and want. You will experience the peace of mind that comes when you know your practice is running smoothly, you've got money in the bank, your retirement is fully funded, and you can do pretty much anything you desire.

Above all, you'll have established a sense of trust. You'll trust yourself, you'll trust your team members, and you'll trust the world around you to benefit you and those you love. When you know how to create a future like that—and you'll learn how in these pages—you'll be able to create great things for yourself and then keep them alive without having to sabotage them, because you'll know you deserve that success.

In reality, many doctors are just like Tom—they feel deeply uncomfortable for reasons they cannot recognize. They hit what I call the "deserve line" (see exhibit A), that invisible barrier that says, "You are not entitled, you are not worthy." It's almost as though they've come up against an invisible electrified fence—it's literally shocking to experience success, and it throws them right back into that sense of failure, poverty thinking, and low Deserve Level. People will then make excuses, blaming outside factors instead of their own negative thought patterns as the causes for their failures. I hear over and over again from doctors, "In this economy…" and then they go on to tell me that it's impossible for a doctor to make a good living in times like these. But we are working with many doctors who are experiencing historic productivity, even in what is being referred to as the worst recession since the Great Depression. These successful doctors aren't using the economic situation as an excuse. Excuses are just well-planned lies. What these doctors are doing is going out and creating more and more success.

EXHIBIT "A"

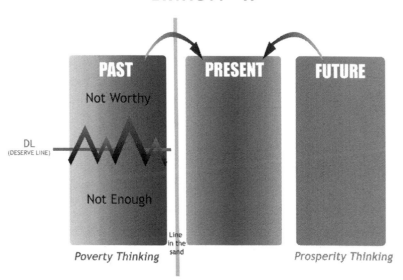

Sometimes I'll hear doctors say, "I have to put in more time or work harder to deserve success." That's simply another justifier, one more way of keeping their poverty thinking mentality alive on the inside, which keeps them from enjoying what they truly deserve on the outside.

There's a distinction I'd like to share with you right now—it's the difference between being deserving on the one hand and feeling entitled on the other. The entitlement mentality is something to avoid. It means that all you have to do is show up and people will hand you things, and you don't have to work, or work smart, to achieve results.

I'm a Yankees fan, and from my perspective, the Yankees had a very high Deserve Level from 1996 to 2000. Since then, their attitude has transformed into one of entitlement. "We're the Yankees, we're the best, so give us the trophy." Sad to say, it doesn't work that way.

I see a strong connection between poverty thinking and entitlement. People who think that the world owes them a living, or owes them a great living, all too often display the same behavioral traits as people stuck in the past—as illustrated in Exhibit A. I hate to say it as a Yankees fan, but there seems to be an awful lot of blame, self-justification, impatience, laziness, procrastination, and self-importance on the Yankees team of the twenty-first century. (I hope that changes by the time this book is in your hands!)

By contrast, when you deserve something, you have an inner belief in your own worthiness to achieve an honorable goal, and you are willing to do what it takes to make that goal a reality.

It takes something special to be world champions in baseball and in dentistry. I believe we are all ordinary people and the achievers are the ones with extraordinary dreams. We are all humans with fears and flaws. It is how you manage them that matters. Of course, a little talent and passion go a long way, too.

People with a high Deserve Level also have a strong sense of responsibility to themselves and those around them—their patients, their team members, their family members, and their world. These individuals are all about contribution. They don't put themselves first, but they reap the success that selfish people can only dream of. People with a high Deserve Level are generous. The more they serve others, the more return they receive. They are open to receive it. They experience an extraordinary level of freedom—they love their work but they don't feel chained to their chairs or enslaved to money. They trust themselves and others. They act promptly and they keep their word. As a result, they have that sense of peace of mind and trust which just about everyone wishes he or she could enjoy. (Picture the Yankees from 1996 to 2000 and you'll see what I mean.)

So what about you? Is your practice just a job where you show up every day? And we all know what job stands for—Just Over Broke. Or is your practice a vehicle for serving others, your way to provide prosperous livelihoods to your team members, and your opportunity to create the standard of living for yourself that you've always desired? I'm not talking about the bare bum minimum so that you're towing the "just enough" line. I'm talking about creating a thriving life for yourself, where your monthly salary reflects a high salary for you, debt pay-down, your retirement, team bonuses, and enough money to do, as I said earlier, pretty much anything you want in life.

The ABCs of a High Deserve Level:

A—Abandon the past.

B—Bail on the bare bum minimum.

C—Create the future based on the prosperity mentality you'll learn about in this book.

When you do those three things, you get *to open up the present*...and that's when you find out that the present moment is a gift that only you can give to yourself.

So why did I write a book that goes beyond systems and scripts to talk about the mindset of successful doctors, hygienists, treatment and appointment coordinators, and assistants?

- Because I want each to succeed.

- Because you deserve it.

- Now find out how.

Larry Laserguy, Happy At Last

ONCE UPON A TIME, there was a dentist named Larry Laserguy whose life was upside down. His office was in chaos, his finances were a mess, and for that matter, so was his marriage. Larry typically carried two $15,000 paychecks in his back pocket that his limited cash flow would not permit him to cash, even though the office was making money. But where did the money go? Considering the fact that Larry was working thirty-five to forty hours a week—not a part of his original plan—it just didn't make sense.

Larry's team was just as dispirited as he was. He had an old-school, totalitarian, paternalistic attitude toward his team members which he sought to leaven with humor, but his female team members often misinterpreted this as harassment. The hygienists weren't happy, because they never had enough time to finish their jobs and educate their patients, which is what motivated them the most. And the administrative team wasn't happy, because they constantly felt forced to do too much with an archaic computer system and with patients who failed to show, failed to cancel appointments when they weren't going to show, and failed to pay on those occasions when they did show up.

At home, things weren't that much brighter for Larry. Although he lived in a beautiful, five-bedroom home with all the trimmings, Larry and his wife weren't getting along very well. Since they had three kids, it was a good thing they had five bedrooms, because Larry frequently needed that guest bedroom in order to have some peace and quiet on the all-too-frequent nights when he and his wife got into it, usually over money or the kids. And the kids were work as well. The three of them were in their late teens, and they all viewed driving a 3 Series BMW as a serious compromise to their lifestyles. Larry drove a 7 Series, they reasoned, so why should they get stuck with something so…entry level? On top of everything else, Larry's wife had been after him for months to put in a home theater and had even gone so far as to solicit bids. But with those un-cashed paychecks in the back of his pocket, Larry figured that he had enough drama without needing buttery leather reclining seats and a movie-theater-size wide-screen to view it on.

In short, Larry might have looked great from the outside, but if you scratched the surface, things were far from ideal.

I'd love to tell you that a dental fairy godmother came into Larry's life, sprinkled some pixie dust, and made everything better. But you and I both know that's not how life works. Instead, Larry happened upon a book. And not just any book, but a book called *Million Dollar Dentistry*, which I heartily recommend.[1]

In *Million Dollar Dentistry*, Larry learned a whole new way to approach dentistry. He learned about how he related to his team and his patients. He even learned about how he was responding to his marriage and family. It didn't happen overnight, but about six months after the first time he read the book (after yet another pitched battle with his better half), his life began to look as if that mythical dental fairy godmother had indeed come along with that equally mythical pixie dust.

First, Larry cleaned up his own act. He learned to treat his team members with respect instead of sarcasm, scorn, and sexual innuendo. He retook control of his finances in the most surprising of ways—by giving the dental hygienists a full hour with their patients, instead of the thirty minutes he had previously allotted. As a result, they were able to do a thorough cleaning, establish rapport and trust with the patients, and then use a video screen (one of the best investments Larry says he ever made) to show close-up photography of specific situations going on in the patients' mouths. As a result, when he came in to greet the patient in the hygienist's chair, the patient was already sold on the necessary treatment.

Larry never really got over his fear of asking patients for commitments—closing cases was still a million times harder for him than actually doing dentistry. But now he had a treatment coordinator in place whose office used to be storage space. In that beautifully designed office, she

---

1 Because I wrote it!

was closing cases with a relish, offering treatment plans and payment plans with just the right language to get patients to say yes.

Larry also installed a new system in the office that provided bonuses for team members based on the cases they helped close, appointments they got patients to keep, and other key indicators of stability and success in a dentist's office. Larry's office was now an upbeat, optimistic, forward-looking operation, one that he, his patients, and his team members actually enjoyed being a part of…even with the downturn in the economy. The team was happy and making more money than ever. *Larry* was making more money than ever, and he was able to have direct deposit for his paychecks, something he would never have dared attempt in the bad old days. He could count on steady cash flow, and so could his wife. Peace was restored at home, the kids were downgraded from BMWs to Kias (if they didn't like it, they'd lose those, too), and Larry couldn't remember the last night he spent in the guest bedroom.

(The office manager whom he thought might have had a slight "embezzlement issue" moved to Argentina, by the way—happily for Larry.)

Larry, in short, was a changed man. He no longer went to work with that pit-in-the-stomach feeling about how he and his team would get through the day. He no longer lost sleep over how they would survive the onslaught of unhappy patients, slow pays, and the dreaded combination of unhappy patients who were also slow pays at the same time. They were all gone, having transferred themselves out of Larry's practice now that he had set in place new standards—pay what you owe when you owe it. Show up for your appointments. If you aren't happy, let us have a chance to make things better, and if we can't make things better, then let's just part ways.

On second thought, maybe that dental fairy godmother really does exist.

On weekends, Larry now had the pleasure of inviting his dental school classmate, business partner, and best friend, Charlie Chairside, over to watch the game in his beautiful new home theater, with the buttery-soft leather reclining seats and the movie-theater-size wide-screen. Sure, you could see every pimple on the rookie pitchers' faces—especially when they did those tight close-ups—but when Larry and Charlie got to see the teeth of some of the athletes, they would muse about how they needed to open a second practice just to help all those players who didn't grow up with proper dental care.

For Larry and Charlie to be friends again was actually a huge shift as well. Larry had grown envious of Charlie's calm demeanor, his happy patients, and his excellent, appropriate relationships with everyone on the team.

Truth be told, Charlie is the one who left a copy of *Million Dollar Dentistry* on the passenger seat of Larry's 7 Series BMW, with the promise to himself that if Larry didn't read the book and follow its suggestions, he, Charlie, would find a new partner.

Today, Larry and Charlie get along so well that on Wednesdays, the day they spend their afternoons in the new dental clinic they built in the inner city a few miles from their office, they golf together. And sometimes, when no one is looking, Larry will kick Charlie's ball out of the rough and give him a better lie.

That certainly wasn't happening back in the day, either.

So here we see Larry Laserguy, DDS, happy at last—his professional life, his financial life, and his family life all hitting on all eight cylinders, just like the latest BMW 7 Series he leased (Larry sure does love his Beemers).

And yet.

Somehow, there's always an "and yet."

Now that Larry's got the fundamentals in place—including a well-funded retirement, something he lacked just a few short months ago—he's asking the question that many successful people ask at this point in their lives: Is this all there is?

Larry doesn't mean this in a discontented, cynical way. He's truly grateful for the changes that have taken place at work, at home, in his bank accounts, and in his retirement account. But now that he's got his basic problems handled, he's starting to think about what else his life can stand for. There are five basic areas that he would like to enjoy even more. They are:

1. PEACE—a sense of serenity in his mind to go along with the outward success he has created.

2. CONTROL—a sense that he's riding the wave, instead of being carried along by a wave.

3. TIME—a sense of having enough time, instead of being strapped for time given his many responsibilities.

4. MONEY—now it's not just a question of how to earn more, but a question of what to do with the abundance he's created. What's his legacy going to be?

5. FULFILLMENT—Larry now fulfills his word, and fulfills his promise to his patients of his office standard: a healthy mouth. But oddly enough, Larry himself isn't experiencing that same level of fulfillment.

In other words, for all the success he's enjoying, it feels to Larry as if he's creating even more success for other people than for himself. Now that his integrity has been restored and his office and home life are functional, he feels he can breathe again. But there's got to be something else left to accomplish.

Larry has now entered the category of what you could call the "successful discontent." He's no longer buying into the negative thoughts, the blinders that many doctors have about their patients or about the world. These include: "My patients don't have any money," or, "People don't do dentistry in down markets." That's all handled. In short, he's ready to play a bigger game. As the expression goes, if your palms aren't sweating, then the game you're playing isn't big enough. Larry is ready to create a bigger future.

Larry has learned a surprising lesson: the opposite of success isn't failure; it's boredom. Now that Larry's got everything moving so nicely, he wouldn't want to admit it, because he wouldn't want to appear ungrateful, but he is a little bit…bored. He senses that there's another level out there—and quite frankly, he senses that Charlie Chairside is already living that dream. But what is it? What's missing? He can't quite put his finger on it or name it, but he knows that another level is out there. The level…beyond the next level, if you will.

The good news is that his old pal Charlie Chairside has come through again, quietly leaving a copy of a second book on one of those buttery-soft leather chairs in Larry's new home theater. And not just any book, but the same one you're holding in your hands right now—*another* book I highly recommend.[2] *Raise Your HDL* is all about finding the depth, the poetry, and the meaning in life that often eludes highly successful people who don't understand why they aren't enjoying their lives more.

If you think about the famous Hierarchy of Needs that Abraham Maslow created, Larry, like many dentists, got his basic needs met with my previous book. *Million Dollar Dentistry* is all about helping dentists maximize time and money. The next step is grasping the concept of HDL. Without this next step, which provides for continued growth and transformation, dentists risk stagnation. The symptoms of low Deserve Level are procrastination, loss of passion, boredom, self-sabotage, and the desire to sell your practice and run away, preferably to a small island in the South Pacific, where there is no cell phone service, no Internet, maybe not even regular phones or mail—and even more preferably with that cute hygienist you just hired.

This book is about finding happiness without trashing everything you've worked so hard to build. It's not about finding happiness outside yourself—it's about going within

---

2 Because I wrote this one, too!

and uncovering the capacity for joy you possess right now. It's just covered up with the day-to-day stresses we all face, and it needs to be freed, like a Michelangelo sculpture emerging from the marble.

So I hope you'll join Larry and me for a new vision of where your life can go. In fact, I'd like you to join me in Larry's home theater, where we've got a buttery soft leather chair with your name on it! And some hot buttered popcorn, too. As you watch the action unfold, a new star is going to appear on the screen—a concept called HDL, or Healthy Deserve Level. Some people, like Larry's partner Charlie Chairside, know all about it.

Now you will, too.

Part I

SEEING IT / *Expanding Your Awareness*

Chapter 1

What's Your HDL?

PEOPLE MAY NOT LIKE going to the dentist. But guess what? A lot of dentists don't like going to their offices, either.

For the past fifteen years, I've been working as a business consultant helping dentists develop successful practices. I chose dental practice because it's one of the most challenging businesses out there. I also chose it because I like to transform people's lives, and dentists don't get a whole lot of love in our society. I thought, here's a great marriage of my skills and their needs, which is what you need to make any practice successful.

In the beginning, I took on the responsibility of helping dentists get their time and money handled, and I naively thought that was what would make the difference for them. If I got their businesses handled and their personal finances straightened out and their time management issues dealt with, if I helped them hire and retain great teams so that the entire practice was producing great results, then surely the dentists wouldn't have to do these things themselves. They'd be happier, and so would everyone around them—their team members, their spouses, their children. Everyone would be holding hands and singing Kumbaya, right? Wrong. I found that out early on.

So I thought, what's really going on here? I'm really good at transforming businesses by doubling and tripling gross income, and I also do pretty well getting teams to be happy and getting clients to be happy. But there was still something missing. The question I kept asking myself was: why can't I take these hard-working, successful dentists and transform them into happy campers?

Then I realized I was transforming their practices and their teams, but I wasn't transforming the dentists' *thinking*. I came to realize that how you think dictates how you speak and what you do. I was so wrapped up in what the dentists were doing that I wasn't paying as much attention to what they were saying, and as a result, I had even less of an idea about what they were thinking. One day I experienced a breakthrough awareness that people's actions—and therefore their results—always march in exact lockstep with their beliefs about what they deserve.

It's not true that in life, you get what you deserve.

Instead, you get what you *think* you deserve. Nothing more, nothing less.

If you truly think that you deserve a high income and a large net worth, that's what you will have. If you don't think you deserve those things, you can work just as hard or even ten times harder than the next person, and you'll still come up short.

The same thing is true with having a healthy, attractive body. If you think you deserve it, you'll have it. If you don't think you deserve it, you won't, no matter how many hours you labor in the gym, or how carefully you count your calories. Just ain't gonna happen.

The same goes for having a great relationship. Think you deserve one? Then you'll have one. Think you don't? Then you won't.

The breakthrough in my thinking was simply this: We have exactly what we think we deserve.

So success doesn't come from working harder, or working smarter, or working around the clock, or working just four hours a week. Success comes from thinking that you deserve success. And that's when I came up with the concept of the Healthy Deserve Level, which is what this book is all about.

A Healthy Deserve Level is a state where you think that you deserve a nice life, however you define a nice life. It could be living in a beautiful home in a great neighborhood. It could be having a great relationship with your spouse and children. It could be success in the workplace. It could be a big bank account. Or it could be all of these things.

In my consulting work with dentists, we talk about how the standard they want to create for their patients is a "healthy mouth." When you go to the doctor for a checkup, you want the doctor to tell you that your body is healthy and strong. When you go to your finance advisor, you want to hear that your portfolio is healthy.

But we've never viewed our lives in terms of a Healthy Deserve Level…until now.

Want a quick barometer of where your Deserve Level is? Look around your life. Whatever you have is what you think you're entitled to. Nothing more, nothing less.

One of the most exciting movies in recent years is, of course, *The Secret*. The secret of *The Secret* is the law of attraction—whatever you talk about, you attract. But going beyond the secret of *The Secret* to the *real* secret of life…if you don't allow yourself to deserve something, you're not going to be able to think about it. If you don't think about it, you won't talk about it. If you don't talk about it, it's never going to materialize in your life. And that's because you'll have never taken the actions necessary to make it happen.

Everybody's focused on what they're going to do next. I want to know what you're going to think about next, because that tells me what's going to happen next in your life.

When JFK said that America was going to put a man on the moon by the end of the 1960s, he didn't know how we were going to do that. He didn't know what actions were necessary to take, and there might not have been a space scientist in the entire United States who knew, the day Kennedy gave that speech, what needed to be done. But JFK, speaking for America, believed that we as a society *deserved* to put a man on the moon.

And we did.

Roger Bannister was a medical student who ran during his lunch hour and set the goal of breaking the four-minute mile. Of course, back then, everybody said that a human being couldn't run a mile in under four minutes. It was never going to happen. Bannister proved them wrong.

Why? Because he took the actions necessary to run a sub-four-minute mile. He trained during his lunch hour because that was the only time he could find in his busy med school schedule. Why did he take those actions? Because he *thought* that he was capable of running that quickly. In his mind, he deserved to run that quickly—and he succeeded. Roger Bannister had a Healthy Deserve Level when it came to running the four-minute mile. When you look at the rest of his life, it appears he had that same high HDL across the board. He was a successful physician in London for decades, and his family life was successful as well.

You get what you think you deserve, because what you think about dictates what you say and what you do. If you

CHANGE BEGINS WITH YOUR THINKING

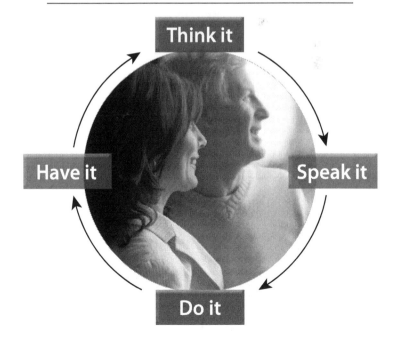

don't believe you deserve something, it's never going to happen because we don't like to be wrong about our own personal beliefs. In fact you'll do everything in your power to sabotage the possibility of getting what you want. It's perverse, but it's human nature.

I believe HDL is the critical piece in the discussion about how to get what you want, mostly because it's always been such a blind spot for people. We all want to have great relationships; strong, healthy, attractive bodies; more money; more time; and more freedom. I'm no different from anyone else in those regards. But back in the day, I didn't think I was entitled to make a lot of money in a short amount of time. It just wasn't in my realm of deserve. So I created my business in such a way that I would have to work extremely hard to justify the income I was earning—until I finally thought I was just going to explode. Back then, I couldn't get where I wanted to go because my belief about what I deserved was so poor. I didn't think I deserved free time, freedom to be with my family, or a lot of money in a short amount of time.

Today, I've transformed my thinking, and I've transformed my Deserve Level to the point where I now have an HDL that allows me to have both money and time. In *Million Dollar Dentistry,* I outlined how dentists can structure their practice to maximize their time and money. You don't have to choose between work and financial success on the one hand and a successful marriage and family on the other. If you deserve it, you can have it. That's true whether you're a dentist, a dental hygienist, or anyone else in your office…or on the planet.

The key to HDL is that we all want to feel good. That's ultimately what we want. We want to feel good about the money we make. We want to feel good about the career we build. We want to feel good about our relationships. It's all ultimately about feeling good. That's why HDL is so critical, because if you feel good about yourself, if you feel that you deserve things…they'll come to you.

You may be thinking this sounds too simple. But that's just your ego telling you that you don't deserve the benefits of what I'm going to share with you in this book!

So the next question is: Why doesn't everyone have a high HDL?

Maybe you were raised by people who modeled a low HDL for you. Of course it's all too easy to play the blame game. I'm going to share with you now what I've discovered to be the number one reason why people have a low HDL. It's got nothing to do with what happened when they were growing up. It all comes down to this: How's your integrity? If your integrity checks out, your HDL will be high. Integrity is like being pregnant—either you are pregnant or you aren't. There is no gray area, right? Nobody's "a little bit pregnant." Similarly, if you act in a manner not in keeping with your integrity, like having sexual relationships outside of marriage or cheating in your financial life, you're going to pay a price for it. Maybe not in divorce court, and maybe not with the IRS. But you'll pay for it in the corner of your mind where your HDL lives.[1]

Low integrity creates a downward spiral in your HDL. Or, to put it more positively, your HDL is directly related to your ability to have impeccable integrity. We'll talk more

---

1 As the expression goes, "The sins we do by two and two we pay for one by one."

about integrity later in the book, but here's the question I want to ask right now: Is there any area of your life that you can point to where you realize that integrity is missing?

If you want the short course of HDL, just stop doing whatever that thing is that you know is outside of your agreements with self, others, and your morals and values. Your HDL moves in lockstep with your integrity. That's the simplest, clearest explanation for why people have low HDL. There's more to the story, though, so keep reading.

Sometimes your past history does have a direct bearing on your HDL. I worked with one particular dentist who, at forty-two years old, was involved in abusive relationships both at home and with some of the people on his office team. He thought that was just the way you had to be in a relationship. When he looked at his past, he saw that it was dictating his beliefs about how he was supposed to live his life. What he realized in our work together was that he didn't have to have an abusive relationship in order to get people to respect him. As a result, he changed his thinking...which led to him getting reconnected with his true self...which led to a considerable rise in his HDL. Gone are the abusive relationships, and that dentist is now a happy man.

I see so many people in dentistry who look as though they have it all. Great practice, great income, the perfect car, the seemingly perfect relationship. They won the game, but they don't feel like they're winning on a day-to-day level. They live in what I call obligation—they spend their entire day trying to justify their success. There's no freedom with that kind of mentality. These dentists live in a realm of justification, decision, and obligation, whereas if they were to raise their HDLs, they'd be living in a world of peace, freedom, and choice.

By and large, these people are no strangers to personal development and hiring coaches and personal consultants. They've done Tony Robbins. They've watched *The Secret*. They've read all the books. They've got the toys… but they don't have time to play with them. They've got the romantic partner…but they don't have the mental space to really be intimate with that person. Instead of feeling free and empowered, they feel plateaued in life (plateau is just a fancy word for rut), and they feel like there's got to be something more out there.

They're right. It's HDL. These people are so focused on winning the game, they don't even realize that they've already won!

Imagine a NASCAR race where the winning car ignores the checkered flag and continues to hurdle around the racetrack at 200 miles an hour, even though all the other competitors have packed up their cars and their trailers and helicoptered away from the track to their next destination. All the pit crew members have gone away, and the crowd in the stands has driven home. Yet, here's this one lone race car, passing turn one, turn two, turn three, turn four, endlessly, until he finally smacks into the wall or runs out of gas.

He won, but he didn't realize he won.

He didn't think he won.

Because he didn't think he deserved to win.

That's the tragedy of low HDL—you already won, but you didn't look up to see that checkered flag. Instead, your life feels like you're just spinning around that track, and you don't know what to do next.

You can't earn your way into a high HDL. You can't love your way into a high HDL. You can't diet and exercise your way into a high HDL. That's putting the cart before the horse. The end game is what you do, because that's what gets you what you want. But the beginning—the place to put your efforts—depends on how you think about what you deserve, because again, that dictates what you declare to the world and what you actually do.

HDL is what I call Radical Common Sense. Life is so brutally simple that we actually have to work hard to make it simple. You've probably tried many things to get there, wherever "there" is for you. We've all been that driver going around and around in our business, our finances, our health, our relationships. In my line of work, I've had many realizations about this, so I'm going to cut the curve on this thing. You don't have to go to a four-day seminar and clap your hands until two in the morning. You don't have to attend a workshop and do trust falls all afternoon. You don't have to do anything. Just stay focused on your HDL, your Healthy Deserve Level, and at some point you'll get it—hopefully before you finish this book.

There's a big difference in life between pain and suffering. Pain is mandatory, and suffering is optional. Pain is what happens. Suffering is what happens when you stay stuck in the thing that happened. HDL cannot do anything about pain, because that's a necessary part of life. Indeed, pain is the touchstone of all spiritual growth. But suffering?

That's needless, and it's pointless, and it gets you nothing more than a martyr's star, which nobody wants to hear about. Your suffering will decrease in direct proportion to the increase in your HDL. Low HDL, suffer a lot. High HDL, stop suffering altogether.

There's an online seller of shoes and other high-end luxury goods called zappos.com. They've got a brilliant way of determining who really believes they deserve to work for that company…and who doesn't. After their training program, they offer each new hire $1,000 to go away. Here's a thousand bucks—now go away. If people bite at the thousand, they were never committed to the company in the first place. Keeping them there would cost much more than $1,000 if they're under your roof and under your payroll. Zappos.com only wants people to work there who believe they deserve to work for such a great company.

At Disney, they say the same thing. Disney spends a fortune training its employees, many of whom will only stay with the company for a few months or years. People ask the executives, "Isn't it expensive to train people and have them leave?" The folks at Disney always respond, "It's a lot cheaper than not training them and having them stay."

If I could, I'd offer you a thousand dollars to quit reading this book right now. Because that would tell both of us all we need to know about your Deserve Level. If you think you deserve to have a higher Deserve Level, then you won't take the $1,000. You'll stay with me, and you'll see what it means to attain a Healthy Deserve Level. If you're not onboard, again, that's just your ego negating everything I'm telling you. "Oh, what does he know?" says your firebrand ego. "He only works with dentists in the areas of money and time! What does he know about what I think I deserve?"

I know a little bit. I've overcome personal obstacles. I went from being a person who couldn't be in a steady relationship to someone who is in a great marriage. My wife and I are successfully raising a child diagnosed with autism. I've had the same personal, family, and business struggles that anyone has who's living life "in the arena" instead of on the sidelines. Today my own HDL evidences itself in the fact that I know I deserve to have only the best clients. All my clients are respectful. They are appreciative. They listen. They follow through on what I offer. Back when I started my consulting practice, my HDL was so low that I would take on anyone. If you had a checkbook and a pulse, you could be my client. This meant I ended up taking on abusive clients who would just keep me up at night—renting space in my head, as the expression goes. They're gone now, presumably bothering some other consultant with a low HDL! So, I am extremely grateful.

People with high HDLs have complaint-free lives. They set their lives up in such a manner that they're only surrounded by other people with high HDLs, people who are respectful and fun to be with. It's true no matter what you're selling. You've got great patients, and you've got others whom you might wish, again in the words of Disney, "would find their happiness elsewhere." Well, as long as you find happiness in letting them torment you, they're going to stick around! A high HDL is the greatest cure there is for the unpleasant or annoying patient.

So how do you think about HDL, anyway? Think of your life as a container. The bigger the container, the bigger your life. Leaks in the bottom of your container? Those are integrity leaks. Better patch them up. Low HDL means having a small container. Raising your HDL means increasing the size of your container, to the point where you're comfortable with having all kinds of great things, people, and experiences in your life. The healthy, fit physique. The great relationship. Money in the bank. Whatever you consider success, it's yours for the taking…as long as it's yours for the thinking about first.

How do you make your container bigger? Well, we've got a whole book to talk about that subject, but I'll give you one example. I had a client who could not go beyond a certain point in his financial life. He didn't think he deserved a certain amount of money that other dentists charged for the same service. So I asked him to look back on his life. "When was the first time you got paid for something you did?" I asked.

"I shoveled snow from my neighbor's driveway," he said. "I came home and was so excited that I got paid for something! I showed my mother the $20 bill and she said, 'Go give that money back to the neighbor. You don't deserve that.'"

Obviously, that moment had a deep impact on my client. He was fifty-four years old at the time we were working together. Because that moment had had such a profound effect on his ability to charge for things in life, he went back years later and asked his mother why she told him to return the money. His mother told the truth, and it blew him away. "Son," she admitted, "I had to give that money back because I owed that woman money."

Was there a moment in your life when you got a message that wasn't congruent with the idea of a high HDL? Was there a moment in your life when you gave yourself that message? How exciting and exhilarating will it be for you to transform those memories, to take away their power, once and for all, and to get to a place where they no longer dominate your thinking?

You are entitled to a fulfilled life, a connected life, a fun life, and a life of freedom—every one of those things and all at the same time. I say you *can* get all your ducks in a row. You no longer have to have a life that's too big for your container, so that the good things you get just go sloshing out over the top the minute they arrive. You've already won the race. It's time to look up and notice the checkered flag that you missed.

I'm not talking about getting fancy cars or a big bank account just to fill a sense of inadequacy. I'm talking about *knowing* that you are world-class, that your appearance is world-class, that everything you come in contact with is world-class, and that everyone in your personal and professional life is world-class because you deserve nothing less.

Let's look at a different driving metaphor. On the freeway, if you drive too slowly, you annoy the other drivers—and put yourself at risk. That's coming from fear. But if you're driving 85 or 90, weaving in and out of traffic, you're putting other drivers at risk. That's greedy behavior, when you think about it—all you care about is your own situation and no one else's. So, on the freeway, if you're driving about 65 or 70 miles an hour, you're cruising. You're doing fine, and you'll get where you want to go in a reasonable amount of time.

Let's say that you want to get where you're going…in an *UNREASONABLE* amount of time. Well, I have good news. You've heard of the diamond lane? In the West, that's what they call the carpool lane. Well, I have an even better lane for you…the high HDL Lane! You can go as fast as you desire. It's the autobahn of personal growth. And you're not putting anyone else at risk by driving that fast…because everyone in the high HDL lane is redlining, too!

You deserve to get where you want to go quickly and easily. More to the point, you deserve to be *world-class*, which I define as *impeccable*. Look up impeccable in the dictionary and you'll find the words "flawless" and "faultless." I'm not saying you have to be flawless or faultless to be world-class. But you do have to establish and maintain a very high standard of what you expect from yourself…and just as important, a very high standard of what you believe you deserve from the world.

Once we raise your HDL, you'll begin to enjoy a life beyond your wildest imaginings.

Why not?

You deserve it!

HDL Highlights

- How you *think* dictates how you speak and what you do.

- It's not true that in life you get what you deserve; instead, you get what you *think* you deserve.

- Healthy Deserve Level is a mental state where you think that you deserve a nice life.

- If you feel good about yourself, and if you feel that you deserve things, they'll come to you.

- You don't have to do anything—just stay focused on your HDL, and you'll get it.

- Raising your HDL means increasing the size of your container to the point where you're comfortable with having all kinds of great things, people, and experiences in your life.

- Whatever you consider success, it's yours for the taking…as long as it's yours for the thinking about first.

■ Chapter 1 Exercise / **What's Your HDL?**

Honesty is key. Answer the following questions by circling the answer (Agree or Disagree) that FIRST comes to mind.

This exercise is designed to reveal the body of work that needs to be done. It offers no clinical implications.

A healthier Deserve Level begins right here, right now. By establishing your status, you can better create an action plan to achieve HDL.

SPIRITUALITY

1. I am living life in congruence with my priorities.
    Agree   *Disagree*

2. I know who I am, where I came from, and where I am going.
    Agree   *Disagree*

3. I have found my life's purpose.
    Agree   *Disagree*

4. There is a great void in my life.
    Agree   *Disagree*

FINANCES AND WORK

5. My financial needs are being met.
    Agree   *Disagree*

6. I am more than satisfied with my job.
    Agree   *Disagree*

7. My financial status causes anxiety.
    Agree   *Disagree*

8. I have a career path that is congruent with my financial goals.
    Agree   *Disagree*

ENVIRONMENT AND RELATIONSHIPS

9. I live in a rewarding environment.
     Agree   *Disagree*

10. I isolate myself from others.
     Agree   *Disagree*

11. I am surrounded by people who support and appreciate me.
     Agree   *Disagree*

12. I am open and honest with others.
     Agree   *Disagree*

LOVE AND SELF-WORTH

13. I have the ability to love and be loved.
     Agree   *Disagree*

14. I am intimate with others.
     Agree   *Disagree*

15. I am a respectable, responsible person.
     Agree   *Disagree*

16. If people really knew me, they would shun me.
     Agree   *Disagree*

ENERGY

17. I am able to identify how I feel.
     Agree   *Disagree*

18. The grass is greener on the other side.
     Agree   *Disagree*

19. Life is full of opportunities.
     Agree   *Disagree*

20. I am empowered.
     Agree   *Disagree*

After completing the exercise, are you more able to target specific opportunities for improvement? Are there particular areas of your life where you feel more or less satisfied? Take a moment to reflect on what you have learned about yourself. Then, fill out the implementation action plan that will allow you to strategically implement change.

▧ IMPLEMENTATION ACTION PLAN

Spirituality
What I'll do: _____

_____

With whom I'll do it:_____

_____

By when I'll do it:_____

_____

Finance and Work
What I'll do: _____

_____

With whom I'll do it:_____

_____

By when I'll do it:_____

_____

Environment and Relationships
What I'll do: _____

_____

With whom I'll do it:_____

_____

By when I'll do it:_____

_____

Love and Self-Worth
What I'll do: _____

_____

With whom I'll do it: _____

_____

By when I'll do it: _____

_____

Energy
What I'll do: _____

_____

With whom I'll do it: _____

_____

By when I'll do it: _____

_____

Getting Clear on What You Want

REMEMBER THE DAYS BEFORE Plasma screens and LCD HDTVs? Remember the televisions with tubes, vertical and horizontal holds, and color tuning? In order to get a clear picture, you actually had to get up off the couch and work the vertical hold to bring the picture from left to right, then work the horizontal hold to manage the picture up and down, then tweak the color knob to get the picture just right. Today, crystal clear high-definition is just an on/off switch away—thank goodness. However, running and managing your dental practice—or for that matter, your life—can be just as challenging as getting a clear picture on one of those archaic television sets. How do you gain a clear picture for your life? Can you see it? What does it look like? Does the picture need some tweaking? Let's take a look.

Goal setting is great. Whether you're creating New Year's resolutions, getting pumped up at a seminar, or writing down goals and putting them on an index card to carry in your wallet or purse, I'm all for it. There's only one problem.

Goals don't work.

We all know about how quickly New Year's resolutions melt away, and we've all been to or heard about seminars where everybody has a really great rah-rah feeling that dissipates within days, or even hours, along with the commitment to the new goals we set. Even the index cards don't typically last long—they get bent and dirty and eventually thrown away, once the person carrying them gets sufficiently frustrated by the fact that it just isn't working. So obviously there's something missing when it comes to setting goals.

I've come to realize that for most people, goals, even noble and appropriate ones, are "should do" things. As in, "I should quit smoking. I should lose weight. I should do this. I should do that." Even goal-setting itself becomes a should—as in, I should set goals!

Why don't goals work? Often, goals are really "because" things. As in, "I should do this *because* of that. Or I need to do this *because* of something else." When you start getting into "because-ing" your whole life, you're not really operating on your own volition. You're not doing what you want. Instead, you're doing what others think you ought to do. Whether it's the committee in your head, your parents' voices, or just societal pressure, it's all too easy to "because" your way into a goal that you "should" accomplish…a goal that really wasn't in your heart in the first place. So getting clear about what you want is the key, not simply setting goals.

It's all about separating from the past in order to invent what you want right now. In this chapter, I want to introduce you to the idea of creating an exciting future for yourself, a big, audacious, juicy future that really fires you up. It's not something attached to the past; it's not related to shoulds, becauses, or other people's opinions of how your life ought to go. Instead, it's all about the outcome *you* want…and how to go about getting it.

I first identified this concept when working with my dental clients. As a business and team development specialist for dentists, the first question I'm supposed to ask is, "What's the outcome you want? Where do you want to get to?" I quickly realized that my clients couldn't figure out what was in their hearts, because they were so attached to creating goals that were attached to shoulds and becauses that came from pretty much anywhere except deep in their own hearts.

So I began a process where I would say to them, "I want you to close your eyes. I want you to detach from everything as best you can—from your past, and from what's going on in the present. Just breathe. Be present.

"And then I want you to look out, all the way out into the future, and I want you to look back from the end of your life."

I actually call it the 'end of your dash' when I'm talking with my clients. Your dash, as in the thing that connects the date of your birth to the date of your death.

"Go back to the end of that dash," I say to my clients. "Your dirt nap date, if you will.

"Ask yourself this: What do you want to be known for? Did you do everything that was on your wish list? Did you even have a wish list? Or did you go through life like a pin-ball, getting flipped around by the expectations that other people placed on you?"

The older we get, the less we think we have the opportunity to create and cause things in our lives. What happens is that we get stuck. In order to open ourselves up, we need to take ourselves out to the future and look back, instead of looking from the present out to the future. The purpose of this exercise is to stop the unfulfilling process of coming from our past. When you look back on your life from the date of your death, you're actually looking out over the future that lies before you right now. This allows for the kind of breakthrough, dramatic, sustained life changes that seldom arise when we are looking at our lives in terms of our present and our past. I'm trying to get you disconnected from your past and totally connected to your future.

To the extent that most people have any growth in their lives, that growth is linear. Their Deserve Level dictates only modest improvements. It's when a person says, "I think I'll raise my fees 10 percent this year." Well, what's stopping you from doubling your fees and getting what you're really worth? The marketplace? No. There are dentists who are charging multiple times what you charge to provide the same service you provide. The only difference is that their Deserve Level entitles them to charge more! And because they charge more, they can afford nicer offices, better teams, and better experiences overall for their customers or clients. Why not you? The only thing standing in the way of you charging more, offering more, earning more, and loving life more…is you. So the first thing I want you to do is start thinking about the rest of your life. But don't look at it from today's perspective. Look at it from the very end, and tell me what you see.

When you create a future detached from your past, you can finally say, *"Here's what I want."* It's no longer about what other people want for you, or what you thought you were limited to choosing. It's about creating a quantum gap that somehow has to be fulfilled. If you declare that you're going to create that gap and make something amazing happen in your life, it will surely happen. The best example, as I mentioned before, is when John F. Kennedy told the nation in the early 1960s that we would put a man on the moon by the end of the decade. Back then, a man on the moon was science fiction. But Kennedy made the declaration, and others around him turned it into scientific fact.

When I take my clients through this process of creating a quantum leap, I invite them to tell me what they want to create. They pretty much always say the same thing: "I want to do 15 percent better than last year. If I have a 20 percent gain, I'll be really happy."

My response is always the same: Let's double what you did last year!

And they look at me like I'm crazy.

But as I always tell them, *they're* crazy…if they believe they can't make it happen.

When you make a declaration about a massive shift in your life, it actually creates a quality-controlled breakdown. Now you have to reinvent how you look at everything, and what you're looking at specifically is the question of where your goals and dreams came from. Are they really what's in your heart? Or are they imposed on you by others, often "for your own good"? It all comes down to how you define failure and success. If you define success as going for it, then you can never fail. But most of our parents never had the clarity to tell us that. That's why if you take this exercise and you look out into the future, you're going to get clear about what *you* really want. Your palms might get sweaty. You might start thinking, "I haven't been able to do this before. Am I going to fail?" The committee in your head is going to try to keep you safe. They'll try to squash the conversation of possibility, this huge, big, audacious, juicy possibility that you're going to create for yourself.

You don't have to do anything about your committee. If you stop paying attention to what they say, they'll just find work elsewhere. That's why it's so important to go beyond the limitations your own mind imposes on you. I want you to notice that you can be bigger than your mind—bigger than the committee in your head. Maybe you've never been offered the opportunity to step beyond the limitations you've placed on yourself. Maybe you didn't know that you can experience freedom from having to buy into everything your committee tells you.

You no longer have to be limited by the opinions or desires or wishes or limitations that other people place on you. You no longer have to be limited by your environment. You no longer have to be limited by the negative self-talk in your head. You no longer have to be limited by anyone or anything. Don't let the ANTs—the Automatic Negative Thoughts—ruin your picnic.

I understand that it's hard to imagine letting go of the committee in your head. They've been there for a long time, so they must know something, right? But if those automatic negative thinkers in your mind are the "people" with whom you primarily associate, it's hard to have a life bigger than theirs. You can spend your whole life trying to get rid of them—what I call "kicking over the anthills." That's frustrating, because it doesn't work. The ANTs are always going to be there.

So instead of coming down to their level and fighting them, why not rise above them? You're much bigger than any ANT! When you think about yourself as world-class, it's all but impossible to hear the voices of the ANTs trying to drag you down.

T. Harv Eckert writes in *Secrets of the Millionaire Mind* that people make 20 percent more or less than the individuals in their circle of influence. That's why the rich hang with the rich…and get richer. If you're not getting rich ideas from your committee, you'd better fire them, or thank them for their input and then stay focused on your commitments. Because until you do, you'll be living life at their level, not the level that you can truly attain: the level of your dreams.

The core reality about each of us is that we all have freedom. Yet we get gunked up and jacked up, and freedom gets buried underneath an overlay of regret, resignation, upset, and fear. We stop thinking that integrity matters. Integrity is being entirely whole and straight with ourselves. We're not living with integrity when we squash our deepest desires and dreams. Maybe you wanted to be a photographer and your parents wanted you to be a corporate executive, because that's where security seemed to lie. Well, the last time I checked, corporate executives are either being downsized, right-sized, or outsized.

Or maybe you are a successful dentist and you are happy with your career, but you aren't taking advantage of some of your other interests and talents because you feel that you must devote yourself fully to your profession. An older client of mine tells me that when he was finishing college in the late 1940s, the advice he heard repeatedly was that if he wanted job security, he ought to go work for the railroads. Today he's happy he didn't follow that advice! There's no such thing as security in nature, and there's no such thing as security in the job market. The only real security you have is when you come from integrity. In other words, you know what you want, and you go for it.

It's all about getting straight with yourself, straight with others, and straight with your higher morals and values. The more you can get straight, the more you'll become congruent between your inside and your outside, and the more freedom you'll have to be yourself. This is the path to a genuine life. When you genuinely express what you want to have and what your desires are, you enjoy life as never before. You won't be living life out of a sense of obligation, and reasons, and becauses, and justifications, based on some past that happened a long time ago. We cannot change the past, but we can reinvent our future, and that's how we get clear on what we really want.

One of the greatest sources of confusion in this area has to do with the difference between means goals and ends goals. You might say to someone, "What's your goal?" And he'll say, "I want to have a million dollars in the bank and a really great body." He thinks that's what he really wants. In fact, those are simply the *means* toward attaining what he really wants—security, which comes from the money in the bank, and a feeling of attractiveness or worthiness, which comes from the great body.

Ultimately, we all want to feel good, to be loved and accepted, to have fun, and to make a difference. Those are our real goals. Everything else is a means toward an end, and we stake everything on the hope that if we accomplish the means goal we'll get the end goal. Unfortunately, it doesn't always work out that way. We all know about the unhappy millionaire or the beautiful celebrity who can't stay out of trouble or off the covers of the scandal magazines. Do you want a Ferrari? Or do you really want the way a Ferrari makes you feel?

When I ask clients about their goals, the knee-jerk response is, "I want more money." But what *is* money? It's only green paper. Or it's a piece of plastic that we swipe at the store. If you take a cold hard look at money, you'll see that it's just ink on paper. It's something that gets deposited into your bank, and since we've become so paperless in our society, it's practically just pixels on a computer screen. So buying something is really about moving one group of pixels on one Web site to another group of pixels on another Web site, and you've bought shares of stock, or a piece of furniture, or a pair of shoes. That's basically what money has boiled down to—it's not even something we see anymore. It's just 0s and 1s that translate into images on a computer screen.

So when my clients say they want more money, it's my responsibility to educate them about the fact that what they really want is more freedom, more peace, and more certainty. These are the end game goals that my clients don't even know how to ask for. So they ask for money, because they know that money provides access to other things.

That's why I mentioned the Ferrari a moment ago. People want money because they say they want to buy a Ferrari. Or a Porsche. Or some other luxury car. But do they want a hunk of metal? No. They want experiences, outcomes, adventure, and variety. As I said before: The opposite of success isn't failure. It's boredom.

There are a lot of different ways to create not being bored. Is buying a Porsche the only way to keep from being bored? Sometimes there are periods in our lives when the only way we can justify our existences to ourselves or others is through the material objects we display. When you cross the bridge into the territory we're talking about here—where you're coming from what *you* want for yourself and you understand exactly what it takes to make you feel great—it's no longer about having something to justify your existence. When it comes to a car, it's the experience of enjoying the exhilaration of a quality vehicle driving down the road. That's true in every area of our lives.

The irony is that getting what you want often doesn't cost much more than getting what you don't want. If you're car shopping, the car to buy is the one that sets your heart on fire, because that's the one you'll take the best care of! So it'll run the best and sell for the most when it's time to part with it, because it's what you really wanted. There's a very high cost to settling for less. It's generally not worth the financial savings, because the feelings of upset, defeatism, and loss over the fact that you're doing what you don't want to do will almost inevitably outweigh any financial savings you might have had. Not going for what you want is an excellent example of a "false economy."

An example from my own life: My wife and I recently moved to Manhattan from Arizona in order to ensure that our son Rome, who was diagnosed with autism, receive the best possible cutting-edge care. We looked at several apartments, one of which cost $2,500 more than the others. It was a penthouse apartment with a spectacular view of Lower Manhattan and New York Harbor. That's the one we took. How do I put into dollar terms the value of feeling great every time I push the P for "Penthouse" button on the elevator, enter our apartment, or even think about it? Don't you think the great state it puts me in affects in a positive way everything I do, every contact I have with other people, and every thought I have? All that…and the great view…for just $2,500 a month.

For high HDL individuals, income rises even more dramatically than expenses, as long as the new expenses are connected to the idea of you deserving what you're spending the money for. Your HDL ensures that you will not only create the money you need for the new expenditure, but even more than that. Why? Because you're no longer experiencing "making more money" as "being greedy." It's not about greed—it's about enjoying everything you deserve!

(As an aside, this issue comes up frequently when I discuss with my clients their attitudes toward paying bonuses to their team members. They often *hate* the idea of paying bonuses, because they take the attitude that the team members haven't done anything to merit a bonus. Excuse me for a second...but how would you have ever gotten to where you are without the help of your team members? Even the world's most heavily decorated paratrooper knows that somebody packed his parachute!)

How do you get clear about what you want? You detach from the past, you detach from other people's ideas about what you should have, you detach from your own shoulds and becauses, you recognize your ends goals instead of your means goals, you determine what makes you happiest...and you go for it.

The other aspect of closing your eyes and coming into your future—or as I like to say, looking at the future *from* the future—is to look back on this present time of your life and ask yourself what you want to be known for, what you want to accomplish, and what your dreams really are. As we get older, we simply stop dreaming. My son is four years old and he's dreaming and he's sharing and he's excited—everything is possible for him. But once we become adults, our capacity to dream goes unused. I can't tell you how many times my clients have shared with me how exciting it is to dream again.

So now you're creating from the future and envisioning

a life that makes you happy, inspires you, and thrills you. How fun is that?

Everybody wants to have great relationships. But unfortunately, when it comes to relationships, we spend so much time rooted in the past that we hardly notice that joy is possible in the present moment. Many of us are addicted to courtship, because when you're in the courtship phase, you're all lit up about the future. We're going to be together, we're going to have a great relationship, it's going to be awesome. That sense of what's "going to be" fuels your joy and excitement in the present moment. So you're making plans, you're doing all kinds of fun things, you're all pumped up. Then you get married, and it all stops.

What stopped? The idea that your future could be more exciting than your present. The future is the fuel for the joy in the present moment, and once you've "arrived"—you've got the wedding ring on your finger, you've got the money in the bank, you've been made a partner, or whatever other future you were shooting for—all of a sudden the air goes out of the balloon. Why? Because you're no longer creating from the future. You've achieved your goal and you start to coast. I hate to say it, but you can only coast one way—downhill.

In a relationship, if the future is the fuel because you're so excited about what you're going to do, then keep on putting things into your future that light both of you up. When is your date night? What are you doing on date night? Are you going horseback riding? Are you seeing shows? Are you even just going out to a nice restaurant? What are you doing to keep the fire alive, even in the face of kids, responsibilities, and the stresses and strains of everyday life? If you're coming from the past, you're mired in misery. If you're only looking at your present life without thinking about where you're going, it's hard to find the juice. The joy is in the journey, the future is your fuel, and that turns your present into the kind of moment you've always dreamt of.

If a magical date night and exciting vacations you plan together fuel a relationship, what about your professional life? How do you create a context for your business career?

When I work with dentists, I have to help them see that their lives are bigger than simply working on teeth and gums. I help them develop a wider context, which includes taking care of the patient's body, health, and wellness. Once they create that future for themselves—that they are responsible for co-creating with the patient a life of health, wellness, and joy—they view themselves and what they do in their work in a much more exciting, exhilarating way. From there, they learn how to enhance their patients' lives on a deep emotional level. Then they grow to taking care of the community as a whole. Instead of being chair-side thirty-five to forty hours a week, they are able to make the same amount of money in less time. So now they have all this time freed up to do other things.

You can't play golf around the clock, and you can only go to the gym for so many hours a day. So what do you do to make the world a better place? You get involved with community activities. Bring dentistry to a shelter for battered women. Work with teens at a teen center. Wherever the juice and excitement is for you—that's where you should go. But you don't get your life into a bigger context until you start to come from the future, instead of the present or the past. You're creating a big future, because when you get a big future to step into, you look forward to what you do every day. I call this the impossible possibility. It's true on a personal level and it's true on a business level that when you create a big future, you get excited, and so does everyone around you.

While you're doing this, you may notice that the ANTs—the Automatic Negative Thoughts we mentioned a moment ago—never completely go away. They get really loud sometimes, especially when you're working to get a bigger, more joyous life. They're there to say, "No, you can't! So says your ANT!" They're actually trying to serve a valuable purpose in your life—they want to keep you from being disappointed and hurt. (Just like a lot of parents we've known.) So thank your ANTs for sharing…tell them you appreciate their love and concern…and then get a book of matches and set fire to the little buggers!

Your ANT-hill—the source of your negative thoughts— will always have a voice in what you do and how you live. You just don't have to give them a veto over what you decide to be, to do, and to have. The bigger your HDL, the quieter your ANTs become. And *I* say…that's ANT-ASTIC!

If you are going to create, then you have to do something I call "clearing to create." True deserving begins when you identify and remove all the justifications, rationalizations, reasons, fears, doubts, and uncertainties that we've been discussing so far. When you acknowledge them, you make room for a life beyond your wildest imagination. I have clients who are sixty-seven years old, renovating their practices, taking on new technology, and reinvesting in the future. They're not planning on winding down anytime soon! Their future is forever; their timeline has no end date. And it's all because they think they deserve it. If they didn't think they deserved it, they would shut down and die, or they'd be walking around like the living dead.

Most people are sitting around waiting for their Deserve Level to rise. Once they feel they deserve more, *then* they'll take the actions they need in order to feel good. Wrong! You can choose to feel good about yourself right now. You don't have to have your circumstances dictate how you feel. You can acknowledge your circumstances, but you don't have to be a slave to them.

You do not have to be a slave to economic downturns or financial crises. Don't buy into those *automatic negative thoughts* that tell you that you can't succeed during an economic crisis. During the worst economic times, consumers spend more money on things that make them feel better about themselves. So, as a dentist, maybe you should focus marketing efforts on Invisalign® or cosmetics. The economic crisis will be a good thing for you, as long as you don't shut down because of fearful feelings.

Your feelings dictate what you think about, and what you think about dictates what you deserve. If you feel great about yourself and about your future, you'll think positive thoughts, and you'll create a great life. Attitude comes first. That's because attitude triggers actions. And your actions trigger results. People say, "When I have a million dollars, I'll do the things I want to do, and then I'm going to feel good and be happy." Again, that's backwards!

You can and deserve to be happy right now, even in the face of practically any circumstances. I'm writing these words during an era that many are calling the worst period of economic history since the Depression of the 1930s. But did you know that, even on days when the market drops 700 points, a hundred stocks go up? It's true! Why? Because there are still companies run by individuals who have chosen not to participate in a recession or in "hard times" talk. Lots of people are making lots of money, even when the majority are wringing their hands and thinking about jumping off the top of a skyscraper. (That's why modern tall buildings have windows that can't be opened, incidentally.) Your job: focus on creating solutions instead of problems or circumstances, keep your HDL high, and notice that you will attract like-minded, prosperity-conscious individuals to your practice. These are people who don't let negative thinking interfere with any aspect of their lives…including their need for world-class dental care from you.

If you know that your future is bright, you can love the moment, even if it doesn't contain everything you want. And if your Deserve Level is jacked up, you'll *get* everything you want. It always makes me sad to hear people say, "When I retire, I'll do whatever I want to do." When they retire, what do they do? They play a little golf…and then they die. They get sick and die. That's because they thought that the day they left their job for the last time, they would suddenly, magically figure out everything they ever wanted to do with their lives. I've got news for you: if you don't figure it out now, you're not going to figure it out then! This is the time to create the future that you want, because the future is coming.

I'm not talking about get-rich-quick. 99 percent of lottery winners and athletes who come from poor backgrounds squander their money, because they just can't be comfortable having it. Their income suddenly goes high, but their Deserve Level is low, so by and large, they waste all their money. It's not about hitting the lottery. It's about thinking through what your life looks like from the point of view of your last day on earth. It's about creating that future and building from it, instead of building off the past.

When you're creating that future, though, it's not about simply, "I want to have more money." Great! How much more do you want? A penny more? A dollar more? Or a billion dollars more? You've got to declare with specificity what you want your future to look like. My recommendation is to take your expenses, your debt, and your retirement needs, plug in the amount of vacation time you want to take, and determine your daily production and collection goals based on those figures.

If your mental committee tells you that you're not entitled, fire the lot of them. Remember that you are not your committee. You are the master of your committee. You are the leader of your committee, and you can be Donald Trump in the boardroom with your committee, look them all in the eye, and growl at them, "You're fired!"... right before a security guard escorts them down the back stairs and out of your mind altogether. It's time for you to abandon your committee and replace them with a board of directors—positive thinkers who reside in your mind and are there to applaud you, be excited for you, and help you create the beautiful future to which you are entitled.

Obviously, not all of this work takes place within the mind. You've also got to be honest about the kinds of people with whom you surround yourself. We said earlier that your income is plus or minus 20 percent that of your closest contacts. Your mental state is pretty much the same—plus or minus that same 20 percent as the people with whom you spend time. So you want to take a look at the people in your universe who you're talking to every day, because they can drag you down if they are not on the same positive wavelength as you. If there are people you feel are adding negative energy to your life, you can and must reinvent the conversations you have with them.

I'll give you an example—my grandmother. Twenty-five years ago, I had a conversation with my grandmother in which I told her that I really didn't want to hear her complaining anymore about our family. Practically every conversation I had with her devolved into a series of complaints about what was wrong with this person, what was wrong with that person, and what that person needed to do differently.

"Gram," I said, "I really love you, and I love talking with you. Can I share with you something that doesn't work for me?"

"Sure," she said.

"Every time I call you, you're always talking about Grandpop and how he treated you poorly, and how you have all these ailments, and so on. You have so much wisdom. I love you. Can we reinvent how we talk to one another, and the things we talk about?"

From that day to this, we never had another negative

conversation. Instead, she shares her wisdom with me, she tells me about her garden, she gives me brilliant guidance about raising my son, and we have conversations that really light us both up. So it's time now either to reinvent the conversations you have with the people around you... or fire them and replace them with a more positive cast of characters. Mark Twain said, "I don't need a new friend until an old friend dies." But I've got news for you—if a person is constantly dragging you down, that person isn't your friend! Misery may love company, but you don't have to love miserable company.

So what's the benefit of coming from the future? You actually become fully alive in the moment. You step out and make choices, and in the moment of choosing, you set yourself free. When you begin the process I've described in this chapter, you'll feel a lightness, a freedom, a whole new awareness. You may not know how to get where you want to go, any more than JFK knew how to put a man on the moon. You may not know how it will all turn out, but it doesn't matter, because you're stepping into your own future. You're making a commitment to choose and declare what you want. In that way, you are set free, and the process of becoming happy and fulfilled and allowing all things to come to you begins right here and now. Goal setting? Goals come from your past. I'm asking you to look all the way ahead to the end of your life, imagine your future from that perspective, step into it, and let the dreams begin. The journey of a thousand miles begins with your first step. Take it now.

HDL Highlights

- Creating a big, audacious, juicy future is up to you. It's not something attached to the past, to shoulds, becauses, or to other people's opinions of how your life ought to go.

- In order to open ourselves up, we need to take ourselves out to the future and look back, instead of looking from the present to the future.

- You no longer have to be limited by the negative self-talk in your head.

- Integrity is being entirely whole and straight with ourselves. We're not living with integrity when we squash our deepest desires and dreams.

- The irony is that getting what you want often doesn't cost much more than getting what you don't want.

- True deserving begins when you identify and remove all the justifications, rationalizations, reasons, fears, doubts, and uncertainties.

- Remember that you are not your mental committee. You are the master of your committee. If your committee isn't 100 percent committed to you and your dreams…fire them, and hire a whole new cast of characters to help you make your dreams come true.

■ Chapter 2 Exercise / **Getting Clear on What You Want**

Go out into the future and look back to the end of your dash. Write out your legacy—what will your life stand for? What will you create with the time that remains in your life? Once you've mapped out your life from a future perspective, share this information with five other people.

It's a *Rich* World, After All

PERHAPS THE MOST beloved ride at Disneyland is located toward the back of the park, between the Matterhorn and Toontown. I speak, of course, of It's a Small World, where visitors ride boats through a shifting panorama of children from all over the world singing the classic song, "It's a Small World, After All." But if Disney wanted to take that ride one step further, then the ride would depict successful adults from all over the world— businesspeople, community service people, dentistry professionals—singing a different song.

It's a *rich* world, after all.

And it is. We live in a world of startling abundance, perhaps startling because we spend so little time recognizing just how abundant and bountiful nature is. If you are a parent of small children, they've undoubtedly asked you how many trees there are in the world, how many grains of sand, or how many clouds in the sky. The answer is that these numbers are incalculable, because there is so much richness, variety, and depth in the world. Scientists discover new species every day. From plants to animals, from undersea life to birds in the sky, nature is limitless. And so, for human beings, is possibility. Actually, the only limit facing a human being fortunate enough to grow up in a free society like ours is self-imposed.

Possibilities and limitations are virtually always self-imposed. We absorb optimism or pessimism from our surroundings, from our parents, from the communities in which we grow up, and from the world in which we live. But there are too many stories of dentists I've worked with who grew up with little more than the shirt on their backs and who went on to become millionaires for us to believe that growth and change are impossible. Indeed, growth and change are the twin hallmarks of nature. Nothing stays the same, and nothing stays the same size.

So it should be with your dreams. The point of this book, as we've discussed, is to help you create the Healthy Deserve Level that will permit you to enjoy all of life's bounty and help you overcome the limitations—almost inevitably the self-imposed limitations—that make the difference between failure and success. In this chapter, I'd like to delve more deeply into the concept that most limitations are self-imposed. This is true even in so-called bad economic times like today. It's actually easier to expand in "hard times" than in periods of economic booms, because now is the time when your competitors are shutting their doors, losing hope, and cutting back. Maybe they're even moving to that Pacific island I mentioned in Chapter One. So who's going to take care of their patients? You!

The ride at Disneyland gives one small demonstration of the ideas in this chapter. But there's another icon of popular culture that's even more apt: the movie *The Wizard of Oz*.

Dorothy's journey is one of the most beloved in the history of film. Why? We all resonate with the fear of being far from home and the need to find a path and allies who can get us back where we belong. But more than that, millions and millions of people around the world have resonated deeply for more than half a century with the key message of the movie: that *everything you need is already inside you.*

Think about it. The lion already had courage, the tin man had a heart, and the scarecrow had a brain. They simply needed to be reminded of what they already possessed—nothing more needed to be added to them in order for them to be successful. Consider Dorothy herself. Throughout her whole time in Oz, she devoted herself to satisfying the expectations of a self-styled wizard...who turned out to be nothing more than an ordinary human being. The ability that Dorothy needed to accomplish her greatest desire—to return home—was already inside her, too. She just didn't realize it. For Dorothy, success began when she recognized that she already had the power to fulfill her own dreams. Once she started thinking, "There's no place like home...there's no place like home..." she *was* home. That's when she discovered that the whole quest to accomplish a goal by means of satisfying the often impossible expectations of others...was nothing but a dream.

They're probably not going to nominate me for film critic anytime soon. But I think you'll agree with me that this interpretation of *The Wizard of Oz* has everything to do with the way we view the world. Many of us spend so much of our lives on a yellow brick treadmill—never quite reaching a destination, never quite knowing exactly where we want to go, never really having the confidence in ourselves that we can get ourselves where we want to be.

Many of us grew up with the story of *The Little Engine That Could* (my third and final voyage into children's culture for this chapter, I swear). The prideful engine, the exhausted engine, and the busy engine had no time to help the toys get to the other side of the mountain. But the engine that succeeded was the one that said, "I think I can. I think I can. I think I can." Its thoughts dictated its actions, just as Dorothy's thoughts, once they were aligned with the power she already possessed, dictated the actions that led to accomplishing her goal.

The problem is that most of us are little trains that tell ourselves, "I think I can't. I think I can't. I think I can't."

Why is that? How do we reverse it? And why is it so important to do so?

Let's take the last question first. It's critically important to recognize our ability to shape our world through our thoughts. What we have on the outside is a representation of who we are and what we believe on the inside. We've talked about lottery winners and first-round draft picks whose inner lives do not permit them to hold onto the sudden wealth they amass, and they're broke or bankrupt not too many years after they achieve their windfall. While these are extreme examples, the simple fact is that most of us—successful dentists included—are and have only a small fraction of what is possible for us. That's because we buy into the mistaken belief that we aren't enough on the inside, we don't have what it takes to succeed, and other people know best what we should accomplish, how we should accomplish it, and what our reward should be.

There are two ways to think about success, money, and all the good things life has to offer. As I mentioned in the Preface, one is called poverty thinking, or lack, and the other is called prosperity thinking, or plenty.

Poverty thinking doesn't refer to how much money you have in the bank. Poverty thinking refers to the way you think about how much money you have, whether it's a million dollars or nothing at all. Poverty thinking is tied to the basic human need for survival; it is deeply rooted in negativity, and even shame and self-hatred. The poverty-thinking person says, "There isn't enough. Or if there is, I'm going to lose it. I can't hang on to anything. Whatever I have slips through my fingers. I don't have two nickels to rub together. Money doesn't grow on trees." Poverty thinking also plays host to a wide variety of other equally negative and self-defeating beliefs—those ANTs we talked about in Chapter Two.

This type of thinking is not limited to the poor. Not by any stretch. First of all, there are countless poor people who don't *feel* poor. I remember traveling to an extremely impoverished part of Mexico where the people had literally nothing by traditional American standards. Yet they were some of the happiest people I've ever met—and it had nothing to do with tequila shots. They were rich in community, rich in culture, rich in connectedness, rich in spirit, and rich in their hearts. They didn't need a big bank account in order to feel the way most people imagine that multimillionaires feel.

By contrast, in our society and around the world, there are multimillionaires who possess huge amounts of cash... but in their minds feel incredibly poor, incredibly scared, and incredibly alone. We all know of Depression-era individuals who grew wealthy and yet never bought themselves or their spouses a new car. Or other people who are so wealthy that they felt they had to spend their entire lives fending off threats, real or imagined, to their wealth. The joke goes like this: "How much money did J. Paul Getty [one of the wealthiest men in history] leave behind?"

"All of it!"

Sometimes even the people who are most associated with the concept of wealth appear to be the most stricken with a poverty mentality...and vice versa. I've spent a lot of time in San Diego, California, and I've spoken to some of the homeless people on the streets of that beautiful city. "Why do you do this?" I ask. "Why are you homeless?" The answer they usually give is extremely interesting to me.

"If you're going to be homeless," they tell me, "wouldn't you want to be homeless in San Diego? You're right by the ocean, it's warm all year around—it's perfect!"

What we're talking about here are homeless people with a high Deserve Level, compared with a billionaire whose actions indicate that his Deserve Level is surprisingly low.

So poverty thinking is not necessarily a function of how much money you have in the bank. I have a friend with a dog who says, "If my dog has one bone, he's happy all day. He just plays with the bone, gnaws on the bone, and he's happy. He doesn't sit there thinking, 'How many bones do I have in Chicago? How many bones do I have in St. Louis?' He's good with just that one bone!"

So you can be rich and think poor...or you can have no money and think rich. Poverty thinking is a function of how you feel about your life. You can feel poor even if, by objective standards, you're super wealthy.

Prosperity or abundance thinking is the other side of the coin. Abundance thinking means that you feel you have enough. It doesn't mean that you're not interested in more! It is just coming from a new place when you are thinking and creating wealth.

Prosperity thinking means seeing the world as it really is—a place of endless abundance, growth, and possibility. Just as there are no limits on nature, prosperity thinking recognizes that there are no limits on human nature. A redwood tree doesn't say, "I'd better not grow any taller than 50 feet high. What are the other trees going to think?" It reaches out to the sky, because that is its nature.

So it is with a prosperous person. Prosperous people reach out to the sky, because that is their nature. The great moviemaker and entrepreneur Mike Todd was famous for saying, "I've been broke, but I've never been poor." Meaning that he might not have had any money in the bank, but he never thought in terms of poverty. He always saw the possibilities in the world around him, and he always acted to make those possibilities come true.

Today, Mark Burnett is internationally famous as the creator of *Survivor* and also the television program featuring our friend Donald Trump, *The Apprentice*. I view Burnett as another example of a prosperous thinker. Prior to *Survivor*, he had been what's referred to as a "serial entrepreneur"—an individual who risks his time, effort, and money on one venture after another, and who views those successive efforts like digging oil wells. Some might be dry, but some will be gushers. One morning, Burnett was reading about a race sponsored by a French organization called the Raid Gauloises, which took groups of adventure-minded types across inhospitable terrain, all in the spirit of adventure. Burnett got involved and came up with a new idea. Why not apply his entrepreneurial skills to the concept of high adventure racing? And voila: *Survivor* was born.

It's sometimes said that rich people spend all their time thinking about money, but the reverse is actually true. When you're wealthy, on the inside as well as the outside, you have the time and space to think about anything you want. You can create anything you want. You can become anything you want. You can study and learn anything you want. By contrast, when you've got very little money, or if you've got a poverty attitude, all you can think about is money—how to get what you need for the day, or how to keep other people from getting what you've got.

Take a look at the life of Howard Hughes. The first half of his life was all about prosperity thinking—he had the financial wherewithal to make movies like no one had ever made before, to date beautiful women, and to build the world's largest airplane, the Spruce Goose. By the end of his life, he had gone from creating abundance to developing an extraordinarily unhealthy fear of its loss, to the point where he lived like a reclusive madman. He was unwilling or unable to communicate with others in a healthy way, and instead chose to hide in a hotel suite while normal life swirled about on the street below.

If you are going to be Howard Hughes, which Howard Hughes would you like to be? The prosperous one, or the poverty-minded one?

The reason we're going so deeply into the concept of prosperity versus poverty thinking is that they directly affect your Deserve Level. You can have a billion dollars and a low Deserve Level, which means that you'll do everything you can to get rid of the money or to make sure that you don't enjoy it. Or, like the people in Mexico or some of the homeless I encountered in San Diego, you can have little in terms of material comforts and yet enjoy a high Deserve Level...and enjoy life to the fullest.

Since your Deserve Level is a function of whether you're coming from a prosperity mentality or a poverty mentality, it's something over which you have total control. You might have been influenced in your past to think in terms of poverty and scarcity. Today, however, you have a choice. When you come from prosperity thinking, your Deserve Level goes up. The higher your Deserve Level goes, the more prosperous you feel...the more prosperously you think... and the more prosperous your outer world becomes. Just as Dorothy didn't realize that she possessed the ability to get where she wanted to go without the help of a wizard, we're the same way. We're coming from lack when we think we need someone else to tell us what to do. When we discover that we already have inside us the ability to direct our feelings, and therefore our thoughts, and therefore our actions, we feel powerful instead of powerless.

We feel that the world is ours, instead of believing that we are at the mercy of outside forces—including the economy. Scarcity comes from the basic, fundamental need of every human being—to survive. We don't realize that we wake up in survival thinking every day. Sometimes I hear people say, "If only I could feel certain about things, I'd be all right." Or, "I just feel like I'm out of control." All of those things—certainty, confidence, and control—are actually choices we make. We might wake up feeling uncertain about life, but we choose to remain in that sense of uncertainty as the day goes on. We might wake up feeling out of control, because who knows where our minds go when we sleep? But if we choose to stay mired in those feelings of "out of controlness"—and it really is a choice to do so— then we have no one to blame but ourselves. Instead we have to shift our thinking and recognize that we already possess the power we need to get where we want to go. We have the power to choose our way of being, and that occurs when we recognize that our attitude or mindset dictates how our days—and our lives—will go.

Most of us get hooked into this concept of "I have to do more, better, faster." As in, "I have to get the next CE credit, or read my next journal, or make partner to make more money." Or, "I have to be president of my dental society so I can have more power and more income." That's what I call the yellow brick treadmill. When you give up this whole concept of doing X "in order to" achieve Y, and just focus on Y to begin with, your life gets really easy. You feel free, perhaps for the first time in your life, and you end up having whatever you want to have, often without the internal struggle and upset that comes along with chasing an elusive dream.

Have you ever noticed that a new employee in the office can be better at a job than someone who's been doing the same thing for twenty years? They come in with a blank slate and truly believe that they can create extraordinary results. Someone could have been doing the same job for twenty years, but that person might be coming from an attitude of, "I can't do any better than I'm doing, and probably no one else can either, so there's really no reason to try very hard." The new person, by contrast, accomplishes more… not because "more" is the goal, but because that person views doing and creating as fun activities, instead of repetitive drudgery. As the expression goes: some people think they have twenty years' experience when all they have is one year's experience repeated twenty times.

So how do you go from being the person who's been doing the same thing over and over again, getting unsatisfactory results, to becoming the person you always wanted to be? How do you move from scarcity, fear, and lack—the poverty mindset—and move into an attitude of abundance?

The first thing is simply to be aware that there is such a thing as an abundance/scarcity mindset. The second thing is to accept wherever you are on that spectrum. Take a look at yourself and say, "I feel like I'm a little bit inadequate over here, or perhaps I'm broken over there, and I'm trying to fix that by showing the world that I can make a lot of money, drive an expensive car, or do something else that looks prestigious and fulfilling." Frankly, that's what I did.

I had a seemingly abundant life on the outside, but I was bankrupt, because I was trying to fill a spirit-sized hole with material things. And it didn't work.

If you ever want to see an example of human beings overcompensating for a negative self-image, take a look inside any bodybuilding gym. Why are these men and women trying to look larger than life? Because most feel smaller than life, and they're devoting all of their time to building their muscles instead of building their mindset. One of the main reasons why people remain in the scarcity mindset is that they are compensating for some area of their lives in which they feel inadequate. But if you come from a place of, "I've got everything I need on the inside," you don't have to compensate. You can just focus on what you want to do to get where you want to go.

People who have enough money, time, and love in their lives are not feeling as though they're trying to compensate for something else. They already feel fulfilled. They're peaceful. They're grounded. They don't live in guilt about having a lot of money, a lot of time, and a lot of love. That's where I want you to go. I want you to get out of the mindset that says, "I don't have enough love." Transform your Deserve Level by knowing you deserve love. And the first action you have to take to support that new attitude is to give away the love you seek to receive. If we're stingy with something, then others around us are just as stingy in return. Be generous with your love…make the first move…and watch your efforts multiply and come back to you a million-fold.

I'm telling you right now: You have the capacity to provide yourself with all the love you need. You don't need someone from the outside to tell you how wonderful you are if you recognize just how wonderful you are. Sometimes I hear people say, "I have too much work and not enough time." That's a mindset. That's a story you tell yourself, but that's not objective reality. The rich and the poor all have the same twenty-four hours in a day, and if you've got too much work, maybe you just haven't learned the fine art of delegating…or the equally fine art of time management! What you're doing in that case is creating a belief that says, "I don't have enough." I'm here to tell you the opposite is true—you have more than enough. You just haven't tapped into it yet.

People think that money will solve all their problems, which is why people chase money in ways legal and other-wise. Yet, if your prosperity thinking doesn't increase along with your income and your net worth, your expenses will go up, too. You'll always keep yourself in a state of "always having just enough," or worse, "not having enough"—no matter how much you have. It's as though a giant elastic band holds you in place. You go out as far as you can, expe-riencing all the success you permit yourself…and then the band snaps you back.

Another dentist I worked with used to have a side business in real estate. He made a small fortune with this "hobby" and began bringing in an income of a million dol-lars a year. As a result, he joined one of the most expensive country clubs in Los Angeles, where he found himself in the company of individuals who made a hundred million dollars a year. (If you think that's an exaggeration, then you don't know L.A.!) Well, our friend went from feeling great about himself to feeling that he just couldn't compete. So he started cooking the books in his real estate company, using money earmarked for one project to pay for the purchase of land to create an even bigger project. Soon enough, he was overextended…in hot water with his investors and the government…and eventually, he went bankrupt. Why? Because his mindset told him that a million dollars a year, a wild dream to most people, was peanuts compared to the people he was now meeting at his club. Did you know that only 4 percent of dentists retire financially free? You don't have to be one of those 96 percent!

I've been in business meetings with bankers whose briefcases easily cost $4,000. Why do you need a $4,000 briefcase to hold your stuff when you could get a brown paper bag to do the same job? It's because these bankers want to display success, perhaps even as an intimidation tool, to others. That's all ego. That's all nonsense. How do you know you've gotten to abundance? You know you're abundant when you don't need to impress people. If you've got a $4,000 briefcase, it's because you really like having a $4,000 briefcase—not because you think other people will admire you or be afraid of you because that's what you're displaying. In fact, when you get to abundance, you actually purge your life of a lot of things. You have no clutter. Your desk is clear. You're not a pack rat. You don't have a garage and storage bins full of stuff you'll never use again.

Abundant people give things away with a generous spirit. They don't hoard things, because they know that when they give things away, things will come back whenever they're needed. An example would be college books.

Why do people keep their college books as if they're going to go back and read them someday? Why do people have bookshelves and bookshelves of books they'll never read? On an ego level, it might be about displaying that these individuals are part of the "knowledge class" and separating themselves from the uneducated. But then you've got to ask—are those bookshelves a collection of knowledge and wisdom, or is it just another way for the ego to show off? The same question could be asked of practically any purchase, from a twenty-bedroom house to a Lamborghini. Why do you need it? Do you have it because you enjoy it, or do you have it because you want other people to think about you a certain way? If you're worried about what others think about you, then you're coming from poverty of spirit. But if you feel abundant and prosperous within yourself, the opinions of others will mean nothing to you.

Sometimes I ask people why they're working, and they have no idea. I had one client, a fifty-nine-year-old dentist, who was successful in financial terms but beaten to a pulp as a human being. This man ran on the energy of fear, which is the most exhausting source of energy of all. His business was a gold mine, but it was underperforming because he had no idea about the fundamentals of his business. He didn't know how much he was producing, he didn't know what his expenses were, and he didn't know what his profit was. He would complain frequently that he had no time for his children, and he would complain that he was tired all the time. Despite his outward financial success, which was considerable, he was living in fear and lack. As it turned out, he had actually set his business up so that he wouldn't know what was happening, because if he did, then he would have gotten off the treadmill, and he couldn't imagine life without that treadmill.

He came to me when he realized he didn't want to run that hard anymore—that he wanted to get off the treadmill and find a better way to conduct his life. Sometimes it takes getting older for a person to lose that ability to run on adrenaline. You can run on it for a few decades, but it catches up with you! I was able to help this client recognize that although he was worth a lot on paper, he wasn't worth much in his own mind. He wasn't running towards success; he was running from his fear of failure. When it comes to that kind of fear, you can run, but you can't hide. It catches up with you eventually, and when it does, there is hell to pay.

This dentist was unusual in that he had a fair amount of money put away for retirement. Most Americans don't have a retirement fund, and those who do save usually do so only because they are driven by fear of financial disaster down the road. Let's look at the numbers: According to the Social Security Administration, 45 percent of people at age sixty-five are dependent on relatives. 30 percent are dependent on charity. 20 percent must still work to support themselves. 1 percent work because they want to work, and only 4 percent are financially set for life and don't have to rely on the charity of others or the government. And a remarkable 85 percent of those who reach sixty-five don't even have $250 to their names!

In other words, in our society, most people are either dead or dead broke by the time they reach sixty-five. So much for a legacy of abundance!

What about the mindset of the 4 percent who actually have a few, or more than a few, dollars to their name? By and large, they're not saving for "a happy retirement" or a "bright future." They're saving for…you know the expression…"a rainy day." Well, if you've got your mind focused on the idea of a rainy day, then you'd better buy an umbrella, because it's going to pour! It might not be raining a few feet from where you stand, but where you are, the rain is going to come down and come down hard. Remember the cartoon character Joey Bifstick in Li'l Abner? Wherever he went, a black rain cloud followed him around. Why wasn't that rain cloud over everyone else? It was because Joey had created it for himself, and he wouldn't leave home without it any more than my dentist client would willingly surrender his yellow brick treadmill.

We are the authors of our own misery. Fortunately, we can become the authors of our own prosperity and success as well. Getting people to surrender the weapons of self-destruction by which they are destroying themselves emotionally is surprisingly hard work. We use the excuse of lack of time, money, and love as a means of justifying why we cannot have more. If we believe that there is not enough time, money, and love for us, then we are trapped in a scarcity mindset. People who feel that way look at life through that lens and search for evidence that they have no time to be right about their own beliefs. In reality, you've got all the time in the world, because you've got the present moment, and life is simply a series of present moments.

We do a great exercise with people who don't think they have enough time. What we have them do is sit quietly for three minutes, so that they get to see how much time they actually *do* have. It forces them to be present. They always come away from that exercise stunned at the richness of just three short minutes in their day.

What are you making with your present moment? That's a function of how you feel about life, and whether you're coming from lack or from abundance. If you feel abundant in the present moment, the universe, God, or whatever you want to call it will recognize that fact and provide you with the outer experiences of wealth—the money, the nice house, the cars, and whatever else you desire. If you come from lack, you'll simply shut yourself off to any possibility that your life could be better.

We enslave ourselves to anything to which we give power over us. If we make money our master, we are enslaved to money. That sense of not having enough causes some people to lie, cheat, and steal on a personal level, and it causes nations to go to war. My goal is to help you shift your thinking, so that whatever it is, whether it's money, time, love, career, or family, that "it" doesn't have you—you have it. Whatever "it" is, it's an expression of the value that you provide in the world.

Why do some clinicians charge a lot for their services, while others, who are clinically better, charge less? The former are coming from prosperity. They hold a healthy belief in themselves and the importance and usefulness of the services they provide. So they feel justified in charging high fees, because they know they are worth it. The latter, plagued by self-doubt, are not as convinced of the value of their services. They're coming from lack—they see their services as worth little or even nothing, so that's what they charge. Which service provider, be it a dentist, a realtor, or, for that matter, a religious leader, would you prefer? The one who thinks in terms of abundance, or the one who comes from lack? Who would you rather be?

We minimize ourselves rather than acknowledging the greatness that we are, for fear that people are going to take shots at us, or out of fear that others will make us feel guilty for being so successful. What does your mind tell you about having money? That you should feel guilty if you have it? That bad people have money? Some do. But they don't keep it forever. As the saying goes, their karma will be visited upon them…but not for your viewing pleasure! Anyone who is successful on the outside has taken the time to examine the rules or laws about money, love, time, and other desirable things or states, jettisoned the ones that were negative or based in scarcity thinking, and instead adopted ones that are positive. If you come from a place of not enough, that attitude it going to run your life and you'll make choices associated with mental tapes like "not good enough" or "I don't deserve it."

On the other hand, if you come from abundance, you'll make decisions based on the idea that you are worthy of whatever you desire, and you'll attract those people, things, and states of mind.

Don't beat yourself up if you come from poverty or lack. That's just the way you've always thought in the past. It might have been the way you were raised. You're not alone—that's how most people think. But here in the present, right now, you have the power to change all that. I want to offer you this new thought—poverty thinking is all about the past, while abundance thinking is all about the future.

In the last chapter, I shared with you an exercise where you imagine your life from the end of your life, so that you can create a future for yourself that isn't rooted in the past. Well, the abundance/scarcity conversation gives us a new way to think about that process. Go out to the day of your death and look back, imagining your future as if you were coming from prosperity and not from lack. What would you be free to create given that mindset? Where could you go? What could you accomplish? If you're free of the worry about how you're going to pay for this or how you're going to find time for that, or whether anybody is going to love you, you've got an enormous amount of energy and power you can devote to discovering who you were meant to be. Then you can actually *be* that person, and create from that positive mindset instead of from the poverty thinking of the past.

Your thinking might have been rooted in scarcity, because that was the mindset of our ancestors going back into the mists of time. Your future, though, can be rooted in abundance and prosperity. You can get off that yellow brick treadmill in which the past keeps rising up to be crossed again and again and again. Like Dorothy, you can get "home"—however you define home—as soon as you realize that you have the power within. It's a rich world, after all, and now it's time for you to claim your share. It is all right here, right now, even though it hasn't looked that way before. It's time that it starts to.

HDL Highlights

- We live in a world of startling abundance. Possibilities and limitations are always self-imposed.

- What we have on the outside is a representation of who we are and what we believe on the inside.

- Poverty thinking is tied to the basic human need for survival. It is deeply rooted in negativity, and even shame and self-hatred.

- Abundance thinking means that you feel that you have enough. Prosperity thinking means seeing the world as it really is—a place of endless abundance, growth, and possibility.

- Your Deserve Level is, in many ways, a function of whether you're coming from a prosperity mentality or a poverty mentality.

- Abundant people give things away with a generous spirit. They don't hoard things, because they know that when they give things away, things will come back whenever they're needed.

- If you come from an attitude of abundance, you'll make decisions based on the idea that you are worthy of whatever you desire, and you'll attract those people, things, and states of mind.

- If you feel abundant in the present moment, the universe, God, or whatever you want to call it will recognize that fact and provide you with the outer experiences of wealth.

■ Chapter 3 Exercise / **It's a Rich World, After All**

Raise your fees...just to the point that it makes you uncomfortable. Business author Harry Beckwith suggests that setting your fees is like turning a screw—when it's a little uncomfortable, you know you've gone just the right distance. Beckwith, however, is referring to the discomfort that your patient may feel over your fees. I'm asking you to do something slightly different—I want you to raise your fees just past *your own* comfort level.

BONUS EXERCISE

How to have it all, in your practice and life.

Step 1: Review and calculate all personal monthly expenses, plus 10 percent—this is your new monthly salary. Pay yourself first, now that you know you deserve it.

Step 2: Calculate your total debt and by when you want to pay it off. Divide the amount of debt by the number of months between now and your end date. This is your monthly debt pay-down expense. Pay this second, after your salary.

Step 3: List out your practice BBM (Bare Bum Minimum). This is your total practice expenses with a 10 percent cushion, plus an average monthly team bonus.

Step 4: Establish a per month retirement amount, depending on your age and the amount you need to continue your life-style when you hang up your loops for the last time.

Step 5: Add your monthly salary (Step 1), your monthly debt pay-down (Step 2), your BBM (Step 3), and your retirement fund (Step 4). This number becomes your new monthly collection. Then pull out your vacation time each month, divide the number of days worked, and this becomes your daily collections amount.

Chapter 4

Your I.V. Is Jivey

WHEN MY WIFE AND I received the diagnosis of our son's autism, at first we didn't know what to do. Drowning our feelings in bottles of wine didn't work because we realized our feelings could swim like Michael Phelps. He didn't communicate, didn't respond to us, and had us confounded about how to react. And then my wife, Judith, got us going. We moved from Arizona to New York, where the best care for children diagnosed with autism can be found. We got him into the best school program for children with autism, we took him hiking every weekend, we got him an artist's easel, worked with him on his ABCs… and changed our entire lifestyle to accommodate his needs and give him the best chance to succeed.

And succeed he did. He's thriving, he's learning, he's communicating, and he's happy. All because we didn't quit.

I'm sharing this story with you because I want to ask you an important question. Are you facing reality…or are you numb and narcotizing yourself from the pain that life often brings in its wake?

Not long ago, I underwent hip replacement surgery. When I was brought back to my hospital room to recuperate, the nurse explained that they had put morphine into my saline solution, and anytime I felt pain, all I had to do was press the button, and relief would come. Even though I had never had surgery before, there was something incredibly familiar about the process.

Suddenly, I realized I had been doing it practically my whole life.

Anytime I had been experiencing any form of emotional pain, I would simply press a button on my imaginary I.V., and relief would come. It was almost as if I was giving myself a shot of morphine anytime I felt the slightest bit blue. Why was I feeling down? The usual slings and arrows of life. Today, my wife and I are fortunate to have learned how to live in financial abundance, but when I was growing up there wasn't all that much money, and there was a lot of pain associated with that as well. So like many people, I carried the disappointment my parents felt about their own lives. Zig Ziglar says, "If you treat all of the people you meet as if they're hurting, you're probably going to be treating pretty much everyone the right way." In other words, everyone's got pain about something. Disappointment. Frustration. Shame. Envy. Sorrow. Unmourned losses.

So what do we do when we feel pain? We all reach for the imaginary button on our imaginary morphine drip, and we give ourselves a shot of painkiller anytime the feelings become too intense.

What's in our I.V.s? Anything that will make us feel better. It might be the fancy new car. When you reach a certain level, the car has to be a $300,000 Maybach, right? Or maybe it's the extravagant house. I've got friends who live in a home that's 8,000 square feet. Who on earth needs a $300,000 car or an 8,000-square-foot house? Nobody needs it…unless the possession and display of such items have a purpose aside from transportation and shelter. But if it's all about proving how good we are by narcotizing the pain that comes when we think that we aren't any good, it suddenly makes sense.

It came to me, as I sat in the hospital room, that since most of us are in pain over one thing or another, we've got our finger on that morphine button—right there on that I.V. drip—all the time. We're all trying to kill pain.

But it had never before occurred to me, while I was in my many years of what I refer to as the painkilling or narcotizing phase of my life, to pull that I.V. needle out of my arm. Face the pain head on instead of trying to avoid it. Figure out what was behind it. Deal with it.

As strange as it seems to me now, the idea of removing the I.V. just never crossed my mind. What's remarkable is that it never crosses the minds of most of us. The national bird of the United States is the bald eagle, but maybe it really ought to be the ostrich because so many of us are going through life with our heads in the sand, not willing to face the danger, the challenges, or the pain of life. Instead, we just hit that morphine drip in our imaginary I.V. and buy one more useless item, take one more drink, try a different kind of drug, date (or even marry) one more inappropriate person, or even just sit there and watch another hour of TV.

We talked in the first chapter about how you're really a race car driver who's already won the race, but having failed to notice the checkered flag, you're just spinning around the track. Now let's shift the metaphor a little bit. Instead of being in the race car, the rest of us are just sitting in the stands at Talladega or Darlington or some other huge NASCAR oval, watching the cars go around and around and around, and thinking to ourselves, "This is the life," when in reality what we're doing is completely escaping life.

That's why this chapter is called "Your I.V. Is Jivey." Because if you've got an I.V. going into your arm, if you're mainlining any kind of painkiller, from compulsive spending to compulsive drinking to compulsive womanizing to compulsive watching-of-*Seinfeld*-reruns, you're giving yourself bad medicine. In fact, you don't even need medicine at all. But that never occurs to us. We live in a society where if you've got a problem, you take something. The problem is that we end up wasting our lives away taking drugs of various kinds—and I include that whole list of distracting behaviors as drugs—instead of facing the real problem.

If you want to find the real problem, look in the mirror. It's not you exactly. It's the thing between your ears.

In the last chapter, we saw that practically all of life's problems are rooted in some belief in lack or scarcity or, in the language we used in the previous chapter, poverty thinking. We've all got this idea that we don't have enough love, we don't have enough money, and we don't have enough time. The commonality between those three statements is the sinking, unhappy feeling that we just don't have enough. Is this true? It's only true if we buy into the belief without realizing we have it. If we believe that life is imperfect and we are imperfect; if we believe that we're damaged, victims, and just no good, then we're coming from that sense of lack or scarcity. We're not talking about poverty in the world; we're talking about the poverty that we create for ourselves within our own spirit. And then we have to go out and narcotize the pain we've created for ourselves.

The problem is that just as the human body builds up resistance to drugs and eventually needs more of the same drug in order to create the same effect, the same thing is true with anything we put in our I.V. If you're making money just to prove to yourself how wonderful you are—and really to cover up for the sense of deficiency you believe you see in yourself—then it's going to take more money next year to create that same feeling of enoughness. The year after that, it's going to take even more. And the year after that, even more still. There comes a point where it can be awfully hard to make the kind of money necessary to assuage that pain without either doing something illegal, or simply working so many hours you end up sacrificing your social life, your health and fitness, and so on. In other words, there are side effects to the junk we push through our systems when we hit those buttons on our I.V.s.

It doesn't matter how nice a car you buy or how big a house you build, because there's always going to be somebody—most likely somebody in more pain than you—who's going to meet you at the red light in a faster, fancier, more expensive car, or build a house right up to the lot line with yours that dwarfs your mini-mansion. In other words, no matter how you play the game of self-narcotizing, you can't win. Your I.V., which started out comforting you, ultimately is going to strangle you.

So *I* say: Rip it out of your arm. Just pull it out. It's only going to hurt once when you yank it out, and for a moment, you'll miss the morphine flow of whatever drug you had been giving yourself. But when you pull that line out, you're going to experience what I experienced when I did the same thing—freedom. Freedom to face the pain, and freedom to get to the other side of it. Let me tell you—the other side is where life really begins. The only way out is through. Deepak Chopra quotes the poet Rumi as saying, "There is a field beyond the field, and I will meet you there."

That's what it's all about—reaching that field beyond the field, where your choices are no longer dictated by the pain. In other words, you get to stop being a slave to the pain and you get to start enjoying your life and finding out what it's really about.

So if all lack has been created in our minds based upon our pasts, and whatever has brought us to that place... and if all life's problems are rooted in some form of lack... then all of life's problems can be addressed by shifting our thinking into a mentality of abundance. If we can create lack in our minds—which is just a myth that we've decided to buy into based on evidence that we most likely received in childhood—then we can create abundance just as easily as we have been creating lack. It's all a mindset. It's all what we believe.

So how do you recreate a mindset?

The first step is to recognize the fact that you believe something's wrong with you. It's about the willingness to confront that cold reality, because so many of us live in deathly fear of ever being anything other than perfect. Yet, we know we aren't perfect, so we assuage that sense of imperfection with the kind of varied drug-taking we've talked about.

I want you to stop thinking about yourself as if you're broken in some way. I want you to stop trying to compensate for some sort of perceived shortcoming in yourself. Because you're not broken, and you haven't fallen short. I've got amazing news for you: You are whole and complete. You are perfect. And you cannot change yourself until you unconditionally accept yourself as you are in the present.

Let me give you a personal example. When my son was diagnosed with autism, my wife and I were devastated. We had no clue what to do, but we slowly pulled ourselves out of the pit of inaction and started to do research, investigate his diagnosis, and accept the reality of our situation. We connected with a specialist, Suzy Miller, and she helped us understand what autism really meant and how to connect deeply with our son. We let go of the notion that we were victims of a situation and instead looked to see where our power really lay. Today, our son is thriving, and all because we changed our mindsets and were able to transform our actions as a result.

Ever believe something that turned out not to be true? I bet you have. Remember when you were in fourth grade and everybody said that fifth grade was really hard? And then you got there and it was fine? Well, maybe you've turned your whole life into fifth grade. Maybe you bought into a bad idea.

Let's turn for a moment to the question of unfulfilling relationships, because this is one of the most common areas of friction, disappointment, and outright misery in people's lives today.

When it comes to relationships, many of us start off in the same place of lack and "undeservingness" that presents itself in an unwritten rule in our heads. This rule says, "I am unworthy. I am unworthy of love. I am therefore worthy only of bad relationships." So we go out and make ourselves right by finding people with whom we will have unfulfilling relationships. Or if a person with whom we could have a great relationship somehow strays into view, we end up doing everything we can to destroy that relationship, because we can't handle the idea of having a good one. What's ironic about going through two or three divorces? What's ironic is that you've been living up to your own expectations and creating the world that you thought you deserved. Every one of your relationships went exactly the way you secretly wanted it to—into the toilet. Now that's irony! And now is the time for the irony to stop.

This may sound crazy, but one of the most common "drugs" that people put into their I.V.s is emotional pain. People crave it. People want it, because they think they deserve it. When you're coming from lack, when you're coming from scarcity, when you're coming from poverty thinking, what are you going to create for yourself? Misery. Pain. Unhappiness. Disappointment. Frustration.

And you'll bring other people into your "movie" to suffer along with you, because something bad happened to you and somebody's got to pay for it. That's the battle cry of the wounded, by the way—I hurt, and somebody's got to pay for it. Not just me, but somebody else. I'm going to take somebody else into this awful nightmare with me. That's why we say that hurting people don't have relationships— they take hostages.

Obviously we're going to stop playing that game now. It's time to stop fulfilling on the insane idea that you are entitled only to bad relationships and start fulfilling on the idea that, as a person coming from a consciousness of abundance and prosperity, you are entitled to nothing less than true love. So go and create that for yourself, okay?

I can tell you from personal experience: You sure can't create love when you've still got that painkilling needle in your arm. You've really got to choose. Either you're coming from lack, which means you need the drugs, or you're coming from abundance, which means that you can create whatever you want, and you don't need to take drugs to make yourself feel better. Again, I'm defining drugs in a broad sense, be it that fancy car, that fancy house, that trophy girlfriend or boyfriend, or whatever else you use to convince yourself that you feel good when you really feel bad.

Okay, now what about money? Not all that long ago, I lost $800,000 in my business. Why? Because I was creating from lack. I was coming from a place that said I wasn't entitled to be a successful business person. Before I could get different results, I had to change my thinking.

I want to offer you a distinction right now—committee versus commitment. It's your committee—that crew of unemployed, slovenly slobs that live in your head and complain about how much everything stinks—telling you to think poverty (those ANTs again!). They're the ones trying to convince you to think lack and misery, and then to go out and create it for yourself. So you can either live based on what your committee tells you, or you can live based on what your commitment to freedom, responsibility, happiness, joy, and self-respect tells you.

What does your commitment say? That you're worth it. That you deserve it. That you might have bought into lies about yourself in the past that you weren't perfect, but you recognize those lies for the nonsense they truly are. Who are you to be perfect? Well, as Marianne Williamson asks, "Who are you not to be? You are a child of God. Your playing small doesn't serve the world. There's nothing enlightened about shrinking so that other people won't feel insecure around you. We are all meant to shine, as children do." Intrinsically, you are already perfect, and when you know that, you don't have to stick anything in your arm. You have no lack that you need to fill. You have only invented that sense of lack and emptiness in yourself as a response to messages you most likely received in childhood.

Now, when I say that you're perfect, I'm not saying that you don't have any flaws. We all have flaws...but we're still perfect, just the way we are. Humanity exists in what I like to call a state of imperfect perfection. Being imperfectly perfect means trusting that all the things that happen in your life, all the experiences that come your way, are there to contribute to you. Either they're making you feel good, or you're getting a lesson from them.

There's nothing wrong with feeling good—as long as we go about it in a healthy way. Destroying ourselves, sticking that needle in our arm, feeding ourselves junk…those things may make us feel good in the short term, but with a long-term cost attached. The real long-term cost is letting our committee drive our lives, instead of allowing our commitment to ourselves be the real directive force.

Getting a divorce? Perfect. If you learn something from it. Business failure? Perfect, as long as you learn something from it. Once you learn that you're entitled to not just good things but the best things, once you realize that you're not just wonderful or great but that you are truly world-class, the world will stand up and recognize your commitment to yourself. They'll even applaud you for it. The world will shower you with all the affirmations that you wanted back when you were trying to narcotize yourself. That's the savage irony of this whole business. All those things that you were throwing yourself away to get—the material things, the spiritual things, the relationships—they all come to you easily and quickly *when you know you deserve them.* That's why I say rip the needle out of your arm, because it's hard to believe anything real about yourself or about life if you're still shooting up.

So the choice is stark. We can go through out lives not feeling our feelings, believing that the whole world is out to get us…or we can look at life as a series of opportunities and contributions that we make and that come to us. Something tragic in your life happened? You're not alone.

Tragedy is one of the great themes of human existence. I'm not here to explain it. No one can. I am here to say that we can reframe our past tragedies and learn from them. Practically any tragedy can be reframed without diminishing its meaning.

Why does tragedy exist? I'm not omniscient, and neither are you. None of us can figure out why tragedy exists. My best guess is that it is a teacher, and that some lessons in life are learned only with extreme pain and at great cost. But again, when the pain comes, we can either process it or we can narcotize ourselves from its effects. Most people, myself included, chose the I.V. But you don't have to. Not anymore.

After romance and finance, it seems that the number one thing that plagues people is body image. We're too heavy or too thin, and in our society, just about everybody thinks (usually accurately!) that they're too heavy. Well, if you think you deserve an overweight, out-of-shape, unhealthy, potentially disease-ridden body, then that's what you're going to create. You'll go on the prelude-to-serious-illness diet, which is available at your local Burger King or 7-Eleven. It's rich in fat, chemicals, and preservatives, and it's guaranteed to take you down.

But if you believe that you are entitled to a healthy, slim, beautiful body, then that's what you'll create for yourself. You'll go on the healthy-slim-beautiful diet, which is available at your corner supermarket. You'll eat healthy foods, and you'll eat enough and no more, because you'll believe that you're entitled to the benefits of a healthy body. You'll exercise, not out of a feeling of obligation, but out of a feeling of gratitude for the wondrously made body that you have. Where do you first create your outward appearance? In your mind. Because what you tell yourself you deserve is what you're going to get. I was able to lose forty pounds when I began to see myself as a fit man.

Life is only 10 percent about what happens, and the other 90 percent is what you make up about what just happened. If you tell yourself a story that what happened was terrible, then it's time to reach for the I.V. On the other hand, if you tell yourself that what just happened was a lesson or a contribution to your life, an opportunity to grow, transform, and be bigger and better…well, that's perfect. That's coming from abundance.

I want to distinguish positive thinking here. Positive thinking doesn't get you very far if you are still coming from a place of being imperfect in your own mind. Positive thinking on top of a negative self-image is like putting icing on pooh-pooh pie. Once you get past the icing, it's the same old, same old. Nobody wants to take a bite out of that. In dentistry, it's like the person who puts veneers on teeth where the foundation is bad. What's the foundation of our lives? How we think. The stories we tell ourselves. So what are we really talking about when we talk about being perfect? What I'm saying is that we have to be perfectly accepting of who we are.

If you have children, you know that they could do anything shy of committing mass murder—and perhaps even that—and you would never stop loving them. You would never stop seeing them as perfect. Perfectly imperfect, perhaps, but perfect. That's how I want you to see yourself: as a perfectly imperfect, perfect human being. As a real person. A friend of mine likes to say that most people think Pinocchio is the story about a boy who told lies until his nose grew long. I see Pinocchio in a different way. Pinocchio is the story about a boy who kept on telling the truth…until he got real.

I'm here to tell you that it's time to start telling the truth about yourself. That you already *are* a beautiful person. That you are perfect because the universe doesn't create junk. That you are entitled to pull that needle out of your arm, because you don't need it, and the thing that you think is bringing you the most relief is actually causing you the most trouble. My friend, your I.V. is jivey. Rip it out. Rip it out now.

Let's take a look at everything we've talked about in this first section of the book. We've talked about the fact that when you have a high Deserve Level, everything you want in life flows your way. We've talked about the fact that most people live in a state of Low Deserve, and, consequently, they create for themselves misery, pain, and unhappiness. This is insanity, when you stop and think about it, because, as we have seen, the world is abundant and prosperous. That means that *you* are entitled to be rich and prosperous, spiritually, materially, in your relationships, in your physical body, and in every other way. We've also seen that we humans buy into negative thinking about ourselves. As a result, instead of reaching for all the abundance life has to offer, we reach for that little button on our I.V. and inject a little bit more morphine, and then a little more, and then a lot more, and then a whole lot more into our bloodstream, without even realizing that we've become addicted to killing pain instead of being free to reshape our lives as we would like. We finally end up discovering that killing the pain is actually killing us. It's killing our dreams. It's killing our chances of being who we want to be, with whom we want to be, doing what we want to do, earning what we want to earn, and looking like we want to look.

So I hope by now you've seen the "it" in this first section of the book, "Seeing It." The "it" to which I refer is a glimpse of the field beyond the field—the reality that our current lives are nothing like what we could make of them, once we quit buying into negativity, stop devoting ourselves to pain-killing, and start living instead.

What does it mean to really start living? Turn to the second section of this book and find out.

HDL Highlights

- Since most of us are in pain over one thing or another, we've got our finger on that morphine button—right on the I.V. drip—all the time.

- If we believe that life is imperfect, and we are imperfect; if we believe that we're damaged, that we're victims, and that we're just no good, then we're coming from a sense of lack or scarcity.

- As soon as you stop being a slave to the pain, you'll start enjoying your life and finding out what it's really about.

- You are perfect—you have no lack that you need to fill. Any sense of emptiness or discontent you have can be remedied. You are responsible. You are in control. And you are capable of making changes, right here, right now.

- You can either live based on what your committee tells you, or you can live based on what your commitment to freedom, responsibility, happiness, joy, and self-respect tells you.

■ Chapter 4 Exercise / **Your I.V. Is Jivey**

What's the hidden prescription in your I.V.? What makes your
I.V. jivey? Maybe it's one thing and maybe it's a cocktail of
inappropriate behaviors, practices, or substances that keep
you from facing reality. What's your fix?

**Write a paragraph about what it costs you to continue to
keep your I.V. plugged in.**

_____

_____

_____

_____

_____

_____

_____

_____

_____

_____

_____

_____

_____

_____

_____

_____

_____

_____

_____

_____

_____

_____

_____

_____

Part II

FREEING IT / *How To Make It Happen*

Be Complete with the Past

I N JUST ABOUT EVERY MOVIE in the history of movies, there comes a moment near the end where the two most important people in the story have a conversation they simply could not have had when the movie began. Back then, they might not have known each other, or they might not have known each other well. Or maybe everything was going fine in their lives, until suddenly the crisis came along that triggered the events that unfold in the movie. For example, a married man has an affair, and finally he has to have the painful conversation with his wife admitting what he has done. If he and his wife could have spoken so directly at the beginning of the story, he probably never would have had the affair.

Or a mother and daughter are finally able to say that they love each other as the mother is dying at the end of the movie. When the story began, the distance between the two of them was too great to have that deep, meaningful conversation.

We even see that magic moment in thrillers, where the good guy and the bad guy have that heart-to-heart conversation just before the bad guy is killed or brought to justice. In filmmaker's terms, that moment is called the mano-a-mano; literally the "hand-to-hand" moment of ultimate conflict and ultimate resolution. It's generally the most dramatic moment in the movie, and everything that happens up to that moment—the whole first hundred minutes of the movie—is simply a prelude to that critical conversation.

In a movie, the result of that kind of conversation is the culmination of the story. We're on our way to the ending, and we can sense that the final moments are around the corner. In real life, when we have these critical conversations, it's only the beginning. The beginning of a new life for both people.

We cannot change the past, but we can change the way we think about it. We can change the way we look back on moments of unhappiness, anger, tension, or distress. But it's very hard to get to that moment without some sort of healing conversation between the two people most affected by it. So in this chapter, I want to invite you to become complete with your past—not by rewriting history or denying that bad things happen, but by going back to the person or people who caused you the most pain and hurt, and talking it through.

Most of my clients recoil when they hear me make this seemingly radical suggestion. And it is a radical idea, because the therapeutic community today usually takes the position that we should either confront our parents or other individuals who caused us pain with an angry letter in which we pour out our feelings, or just ignore them and walk away. I'm proposing a middle path, in which we have a serious, meaningful, and admittedly often painful conversation with the person who we believe caused us pain. Why? Because the more you understand, the harder it is to keep suffering.

In the previous chapter, we talked about how your I.V. is jivey, and that now's the time for you to rip the painkilling medication out of your arm and face reality. In this chapter, we're talking about the reality that needs to be faced. A specific moment from the past. The climate in your home throughout your childhood. A marriage gone bad. A relationship with a parent that somehow failed. That's what I mean when I talk about being complete with the past.

Instead of confronting the person angrily or ignoring the whole thing and wishing it would somehow go away (it won't), this middle path pays enormous dividends. First, you get to gain perspective on what happened, an often extremely surprising perspective that reframes the whole experience in a way that takes away its sting. In other words, you don't have to go on hurting the way you've been hurting, because you suddenly see the situation in a new light. It's also healing for the other person, who has probably been suffering just as much as you have and who would relish the opportunity, if not to come right out and apologize— apologies are tough—then to at least explain themselves, come to terms with what happened, and move on.

Is this going to work for everyone? No, absolutely not. This is a step you might want to take with the guidance of a trusted advisor. It's possible to achieve astonishing healing through the simple act of two people telling each other the truth and taking responsibility where needed.

The problem with the past is that it does not stay in the past. It recurs inside of our souls every moment that we go back to it in thought. When the terrorists attacked on 9/11, their goal was not simply to take down buildings or disrupt an economy. Their goal was to have the emotion of fear recur in a constant basis on the part of all 300 million Americans, not just the families of the approximately 3,000 who were killed in the attacks. And the news media jumped on the bandwagon. It's fair to say that while Al-Qaeda attacked us only once, CNN has attacked the psyche of the country day after day after day, reminding us of the attack and creating a climate of fear—all in the name of ratings. Now the media is doing the same thing with the economic crisis.

What the TV networks do to us in terms of creating uncomfortable emotions for the sake of a financial payoff, we also do to ourselves. But this time, the payoff is a bit more subtle. It allows us to reinforce the notion that we're bad, wrong, inappropriate, and, most of all, that we're not enough. That puts us back on the merry-go-round of pain-killing, causing us to reach, every time we have a painful thought, for the button on our I.V. I'm not proposing on a global scale that the President of the United States sit down with Osama Bin Laden and "talk it out"—although if world leaders could have those kinds of conversations, there might never have been the tension and frustration on the part of our opponents that led to those terrorist attacks. But to take the subject back to our daily lives, it's all about recognizing that if we can sit down with the person who harmed us and talk things out, the healing will begin.

I don't believe in lying to myself about the past. The things that happened, happened. It's said that memories are like TNT—the harder you push them down, the bigger the explosion when they finally come out. So we're talking about serving as our own bomb detonation squad. We're taking that dynamite…and diffusing it.

When we do so, we don't need to stay trapped in that cycle of pain, painkilling, more pain, and more painkilling. What messages from the past are we overcoming? The message itself takes many forms, but the bottom line is always the same: That we're not worthy. We're not worthy of love. We're not worthy of money. We're not worthy of health. We're not worthy of having a life that might even be better from a material perspective than our parents'. Learning to let go of the mistaken belief that we are unworthy, a belief that we most likely acquired in childhood, is vitally important.

But there's only so much that we can do on our own. The missing piece for many people, including a number of my clients who have spent years in therapy or in twelve-step programs coping with this issue, requires a conversation with the person who caused the pain in the first place. This conversation, for some of my clients, has taken place at cemeteries, because their parents are no longer alive. It's best, of course, to take this step while the individuals we need to speak to are still living and able to respond. That means there's no time to be lost in making these conversations happen.

This is how we get complete with the past, and this is how we begin to develop the freedom that allows us to create the lives we truly deserve. It's about drawing a line in the sand and saying, "This is the past. Now it gets to stay in the past. I don't have to take it into my daily thoughts and decision-making process. I can let it go." And when you can do that, you can truly live in the present

Do you know why they call it the present? Because the present is a gift. And not just any gift…but the very best gift you can give yourself.

HDL Highlights

- We cannot change the past, but we can embrace it, acknowledge it, and ultimately change the way we think about it.

- You can become complete with your past—not by rewriting history or denying that bad things happen, but by going back to the person or people who caused you the most pain and hurt, and talking it through.

- Learning to let go of the mistaken belief that we are unworthy is vitally important.

- When you can relinquish the past, you can truly live in the present.

- The reason we call it the "present" is because the present is a gift. And not just any gift...but the very best gift you can give yourself.

■ Chapter 5 Exercise / **Be Complete with the Past**

Make a list of at least five people you have been avoiding or resenting. Then, arrange to have a crucial conversation with each of them.

Step 1: Acknowledge the person and the relationship you have with them.

"Dr. Smith, I really appreciate our relationship."

Step 2: Ask permission to have a serious conversation.

"Dr. Smith, can I have a few minutes of your time to discuss something that doesn't work for me about our relationship?"

Step 3: Address the discomfort, resentment, or issue you have with them.

"Are you aware that… "

- "… when you're late, it sends a message that you don't care?"
- "… you invalidate me in front of patients?"
- "… every time I try to ask for a raise, you dismiss me?"

Step 4: Listen.

Step 5: Go forward with a new agreement. Find a common ground and a plan for the future.

- "Dr. Smith, can you agree to be on time?"
- "Dr. Smith, can you agree to address any problem you have with me in a private setting?"

Once you have worked through each person and each issue or problem, make sure to maintain your part of the agreement. If you notice the other person is failing to act in accord with the agreement, address it and re-work the steps accordingly.

Chapter 6

Keeping Your Word

IN THE BEGINNING was the word.

Your word.

In this chapter, I want to share with you the importance of keeping your word and keeping your agreements. We've spent a lot of time and effort creating a new present for you, one where you are not forced to self-medicate due to prior events. So the question now becomes: How do you turn your present into the life that you've always deserved? To answer this question, I want to talk with you about the importance of keeping agreements as a means of attaining the spectacular life that awaits you...all as a result of your new, high HDL.

It's really amazing how quickly we undervalue our word. We tell someone with all sincerity that we'll be there at 9:30, but we don't really get there until 9:33 or 9:34. We step right over being late and fail to take responsibility. Shakespeare wrote that punctuality is the courtesy of kings, and when we fail to be punctual, we are actually showing disrespect for the time of the other person. And in our time-pressed society, there is no greater theft possible, because a minute lost can never be regained.

Sometimes we fail to keep our word to ourselves. We *say* that we're going to take full advantage of our new gym membership and get there three times a week. Then three times dwindles down to twice a week, which becomes once a week, which slowly slides into…never.

Or we might make a moral commitment to ourselves—we will attend church every Sunday. Or we will quit smoking. Then Sunday comes and we sleep in. And when nobody's looking…we sneak out for a quick cigarette.

There is an extremely high cost for failing to keep our agreements with others, with ourselves, and with our morals and values. One of my clients says that when he was failing to keep agreements, as he put it, "I didn't think anybody was noticing. I thought I was walking between the raindrops, but before I knew it, I was totally drenched." After working day in day out for years in our careers, we eventually get to a point where we're doing everything by rote. We're not focused on delivering maximum value to our patients. We are no longer keeping our commitment to ourselves or to our teams to be world-class.

Working with thousands of dentists, I see this frequently. There are all too many dentists who fail to recommend treatment to their patients, simply because they have been down the road of rejection too many times and they don't want to hear the word "no" again. But by failing to take the risk of rejection, they are failing to provide their patients with what they really need—the right treatment. In so doing, they're doing their patients a disservice, and they are sabotaging their own professional success. Either we're buying into our commitment to be world-class, or we're selling out to the all-too-human traits of laziness, torpor, and low standards.

People are sometimes put off by the word "integrity." It sounds scary. It sounds unattainable. But integrity doesn't specifically mean honesty and truthfulness, although those are certainly aspects of the term. Integrity really means wholeness. When we restore our level of integrity by creating and maintaining good agreements, we are restoring our wholeness.

When we come out of a childhood or out of a bad marriage that feels like failure, we can feel like a dented can—incomplete, imperfect, and in need of a fix. When that happens, we end up coming from effect and not cause. We find ourselves at the mercy of anyone or anything that comes along, and we go through life like a leaf driven by the wind, first here, then there, but never really setting our own course. One of my clients told me about a meeting with two patients, a mother and a daughter, who had beaten him up pretty severely in an effort to get a better price. They had attacked his integrity and complained about the quality of his care. He immediately went into "What can I do to make this better?" mode, even offering to reduce the price if it would appease them. The patients told him that "while he was still being considered," they would have to contact other dentists to compare quality and prices.

About an hour after that conversation, he realized that he had not been coming from a world-class state of mind. When confronted with an attack, a world-class person would simply say, "I won't be able to help you! We have bent over backwards to try and serve you. Thank you for your time!" And the matter would be over. World-class people and organizations don't have to fight to demonstrate their integrity. As the expression goes, what they do speaks so loudly that you can hardly hear a word they're saying!

After coming to this realization, my client sent those clients an e-mail to this effect: "I regret that I haven't been able to meet your expectations. Thank you for the opportunity to serve you. Please let us know where we can send your records."

He sent the e-mail, and he neither regretted nor looked back. When you keep your agreements, you come from a place of wholeness and completion, and that's what integrity's all about. You're no longer causing frustration for yourself or other people through missing or broken agreements. Instead, you're keeping those agreements, and holding yourself and others to the highest standard as a result.

Let's look at the three areas of agreements that we must learn to keep. First, we must keep agreements with others. This builds trust. A client of mine in California had promised a new dental hygienist in her office a review, including a salary review, within ninety days of joining the practice. The ninety days came and went, but there was no review. The dentist running the practice had been sincere in her commitment to give the new hire a review, but she had simply failed to schedule it and the commitment became lost in the usual tumult of work. It soured the new dental hygienist on the work situation, and before long, he left because he believed that his employer had given him a glimpse of the way things would always be in that office. As it turned out, he was right.

Are you losing employees because you are failing to keep your word? The item in question may not seem terribly important to you, but if you give your word to someone else, that other person is going to take what you have to say extremely seriously. When your word loses power, so do you…which means you also lose your ability to expand and make positive changes.

I gave the example earlier of the individual who runs late for a meeting. If you get to an appointment late and you offer a sincere apology or, better still, if you have someone on your team explain that you're a few minutes behind schedule—then you haven't lost trust. But if you act as if your time is important and the other person's is not, you've set yourself up for disaster, no matter how good or valuable you or your practice might be. Lip service doesn't cut it. You've got to keep all of the agreements you create with others, or you will cause frustration and disappointment, which will turn around and bite you before long.

The second kind of agreement you must keep is with yourself. Self-worth comes from doing what you say you'll do, when you say you'll do it. This could be as simple as your commitment to go to the gym, your commitment to lose weight, your commitment to get caught up on your taxes, or whatever the issue might be. In life, most of us get into trouble not for what we do, but for what we leave undone. If you make an agreement with yourself, you must honor it, no questions asked. If you don't, you need to restore your word with yourself and get back on the commitment trail.

The third kind of agreement has to do with your morals and values. If your morality dictates, as I mentioned a moment ago, that you attend religious services on a regular basis, then you've got to do so. If your values include not using profanity around your spouse, then keep your word.

The life that you want to create is a function of your ability to keep your word. That's integrity. That's wholeness. That's keeping your agreements. When you are living your agreements, there's a wonderful side benefit—you get to live your dreams. Failing to live one's agreements is a means of distracting oneself from the major issue of who you are and who you want to be in the world. If money is the only thing in your I.V., you can't really be whole. You're spending your entire day shooting yourself up instead of turning yourself on. When you take care of your integrity issues by filling the leaks in your bucket, you can then begin to concentrate on something that's considerably more exciting—finding out who you're really supposed to be.

Reverend Jesse Jackson speaks of "the me that makes me me." I want to speak for a moment about the "you that makes you you"—what I call your U3. Your U3 is who you are meant to be in the world. It is for you and you alone to decide. But it's only possible to focus on the question of your U3 when you've gotten straight with the past and when you have committed to keeping your agreements to others, to yourself, and to your morals and values. Only then do you get to determine what your U3 really is. When you are living with a cleared-up past and in a state of commitment to keeping your agreements, then you can really get into your U3. And living in your U3...will lead you straight to euphoria.

HDL Highlights

- There is an extremely high cost for failing to keep our agreements with others, with ourselves, and with our morals and values.

- Either we are buying into our commitment to be world-class, or we're selling out to the all-too-human traits of laziness, torpor, and low standards.

- Integrity really means wholeness. When we restore our level of integrity by creating and maintaining good agreements, we are restoring our wholeness.

- World-class people and organizations don't have to fight to demonstrate their integrity.

- When you keep your agreements, you come from a place of wholeness and completion, and that's what integrity is all about.

- Keep agreements with others, yourself, and with your morals and values. Self-worth comes from doing what you say you'll do, when you say you'll do it.

- When you are living with a cleared-up past and in a state of commitment to keeping your agreements, then you can really get into your U3—the you that makes you you.

■ Chapter 6 Exercise / **Keeping Your Word**

1. Make a list of all your broken agreements with yourself
    and others. List who and what needs to be addressed,
    and also list by what deadline you'll clean it all up.

2. Write your U3—your purpose as a dentist, hygienist,
    treatment coordinator, appointment coordinator, or
    dental assistant. Then add the you that makes you you in
    the other areas of your life—at home, in social settings,
    and anywhere else where your U3 can shine.

Freeing Your World

I COULD HAVE CALLED this chapter "cleaning your world," but nobody would have wanted to read it! The whole idea of cleaning sounds boring, menial, and repetitive. But the cleansing we're going to accomplish in this chapter is anything but. It's going to be exciting, fascinating, and life-changing, because we are getting rid of the old low Deserve Level in our physical environment and making space for the rich, exciting HDL environment we truly deserve. There's nothing dull about that.

In the previous two chapters, we talked about the freedom that develops when we clean up the wreckage of our past, first by engaging with the people who might have caused us the most pain and coming to terms with those relationships, and then by recognizing the importance of being true to our word. Keeping one's word to others and to ourselves, and thereby living in tune with the values we possess, is paramount. Otherwise, we're just back to filling up that I.V. with junk. Maybe more expensive junk, but it's the same old junk. As the expression goes, if nothing changes, then nothing changes. Now it's time to make some seemingly small, insignificant changes that will have important implications for the way you live your life.

We live in a time of intense concern for the environment. People are concerned, and rightly so, about sustainability, global warming, our carbon footprint, the ozone layer, the melting of the ice caps, and all the other dangers that modern society has brought to the fragile ecosystem that is planet Earth. We understand that if life is not sustainable, then we can't live in a healthy manner. So the world is going green.

But what about the individual ecosystem in which each of us lives? What about the world we create for ourselves? Every human being lives in a self-created universe, which consists of all the things we use each day to survive, thrive, and better our lives. I'm talking about the food we eat, the clothing we wear, the vehicles we drive, the homes in which we live, and the offices where we work. Just for a moment, let's move away from global environment concerns and let's get local. Really local. As local as the trunks of our cars, or the desks in our offices. Because when it comes to personal environments, it doesn't get much more local than that!

How do you live? What kind of environment have you created for yourself? Is it neat and orderly? Can you find stuff, be it a magazine you're looking for or a particular document on your desk or your laptop? Do you treat your inbox like a safety deposit box, where you keep stuff forever even though it might have no value, now or in the future? How long have certain things been sitting on your desk? Do you have any clue what is at the bottom of that pile lurking on the right hand corner?

The things in our lives, from the stuff we keep in the trunk of our cars (and on the floor of the back seat) to the papers we keep on our desks, speak volumes about us. If they could talk, what story would they tell? "This guy's clean!" Or would they say, "Houston, we have a problem"?

People like to joke about this. They say, "I know they say cleanliness is next to godliness, but for me, cleanliness is next to impossible." Or, "A clean car is the sign of a sick mind." It's funny…but only up to a point. Because the serious point is that just as the global environment cannot survive if it's clogged up with pollutants, excessive chemicals, too much heat, and all the other negatives that modern society creates, we cannot be our best selves and we cannot do our best work if our personal environment is jammed up with all kinds of stuff we don't need, don't use, or can't find. If we are truly to free our HDL, then our personal environment must be as supportive to us as we would have the global environment become. We're talking about HDL sustainability. The good news is that it's a lot easier to establish a high level of HDL in your personal world than for the whole planet.

Let's start with your desk. I am always interested to see the way my clients treat their desks. A quick way to estimate a client's HDL is to look at the cleanliness and tidiness of his or her desk. In my work with dentists, I've found that there is a direct correlation between cleanliness and high HDL, and messiness and low HDL.

Cars are much the same. Sometimes you see cars that are outright rolling junk wagons, usually ten- to fifteen-year-old beaters crammed from the carpet to the glove box with old newspapers, old junk, old everything. You look at the drivers of those cars and you ask yourself, "How could they live that way?" But the reality is that most of us live in a manner more similar to those rolling junk heaps than we would care to admit. Our cars might be a little newer, a little cleaner, and a little classier, but if we are tolerating junk in our environment, we're giving ourselves—and any poor unfortunates who happen to come in the car (or office) with us—the message that this is all we deserve.

And that's a low Deserve Level.

A clean desk and a clean car, on the other hand, are signs of a high HDL. It's that simple. There's something magical about going to the car showroom, because all of the cars are spotless. At a high-end dealership, every one of those cars is washed, vacuumed, and generally cleaned within an inch of its life every single day. In part, "new car smell" is the absence of anything we associate with "old car smell"—wrappers, bits of food, spilled coffee or soda that have become one with the upholstery, and so on. If your car's a mess, so is your HDL. It might have taken months or even years to get your car to the level of sloppiness that it currently demonstrates, but it probably would only take twenty minutes or so to straighten it out.

It's the same with your desk.

Just as there is a huge difference between entering a clean car and entering a rolling recycling bin, there is a huge difference between working at a tidy desk and working atop a heaping pile of who knows what. Every cell in your body feels the difference. It's a small way to tell yourself that you matter, that you are worthy of a nice environment, and that you have enough self-respect to keep your things clean and orderly.

It really doesn't matter how many Tony Robbins seminars you attend if, the moment you step out of the seminar after having walked on hot coals or swum from Hawaii to Fiji, you get back in your car and your car is a pit. There's no simpler way to show yourself disrespect than to force yourself to subsist in a messy environment. Yet we do this to ourselves constantly, giving ourselves a very negative message many times each day.

Right now, I'd like to invite you to take twenty minutes and clean out your desk, and then take another twenty minutes to clean out your car. Those forty minutes should allow you plenty of time to clean out these two places where, if you're like most Americans, you spend a good deal of your time. And don't just do the top of your desk or the dashboard of your car. Really dig around deep to dislodge all the clutter. You never know what treasures you may find!

Once you've cleaned out your desk, the most important thing you'll discover is that you feel good about yourself. So why not go ahead and commit yourself to keeping your desk clean? It certainly helps set a positive example for the rest of the office. What kind of message are you giving your team about yourself and about the Deserve Level to which they should aspire? Sloppy is as sloppy does. It's time to put sloppy to bed and create an environment for yourself that demonstrates to you and to the world that you don't just deserve better…you deserve the best.

By the way, what are you driving? If you don't have a nice car, get one. I worked with one dentist who drove a twenty-year-old Mustang. Not a classic '65—just an old beater of a car. I suggested strongly that he get a car that demonstrated a higher HDL. He wouldn't put patients in a twenty-year-old chair in his operatory, would he? (I hoped not!) Shortly afterwards, he bought a nice Cadillac STS. Not-so-incidentally, his production went from $35,000 a month to $65,000 a month.

There's absolutely no excuse for driving around in something that demonstrates a low HDL. It destroys your patient's confidence in you, and it makes them wonder if you're really the right person for the job. The "millionaire next door" might be driving a twelve-year-old Lincoln. Good for him. If you're not a millionaire and you want to be, start driving like one. Get behind the wheel of something that gives you a sense of self-respect and pride every time you step into the car. Ironically, in my low HDL days, I bought a Porsche, because I thought I could derive self-esteem from my vehicle. Instead, nobody ever complimented me on how nice the car was, and I felt even worse. Today, I drive a nice car—a 7 Series BMW, since you've asked—and I get compliments all the time on it. I don't drive it because I'm coming from a place of low self-esteem. I drive it because I deserve it, and people respond to the sense of high Deserve Level that the car symbolizes.

A number of my clients with messy desktops have posed the same question to me. Without fail, they always ask it in an extremely confidential manner, with low voices, in settings where no one else can hear. They say, "How do they do it, Gary? How do they keep their desks so neat, tidy, and orderly? Why can't I?" I'll tell you exactly what I tell them: a cluttered desk is a cluttered mind.

The same mentality that leads some people to turn their cars into rolling trash bins also evidences itself in the workplace in terms of the desk that ate Chicago. What are the psychological reasons for messy desks? It's got nothing to do with laziness, because some people with sloppy desks are among the hardest workers I've ever met. Instead, it's a hoarding mentality that says, "If I don't have all my stuff where I can see it, I might lose it." Or an even deeper reality for many of these individuals is that they simply don't think they deserve to ever finish their work, because they feel the need to keep themselves on that treadmill, always running faster and faster and never getting anywhere. The desk overcome with paper reinforces that notion of work-as-treadmill. It sends a message to the occupant of the desk—and to all those who come in contact with him or her—that this is a person who just never gets anything finished.

I can tell you from working with dentists that when patients see sloppy desks, they lose confidence. Patients want to be certain that a doctor will always have immediate access to important medical records, and that no vital document will get lost. A messy desk is a way of telling everyone in your working world that they don't really matter, because the messy desk person doesn't consider documents relating to other people to be important enough to file away securely. I can look at a doctor's desk and tell you just how chaotic his or her life is. Are there old, unread copies of *Dental Economics* stacked up everywhere? Old cases? Sticky notes on the computer screen? Don't let anybody tell you that a clean desk is the sign of a sick mind. That's certainly not how your patients see it.

When your desktop is clean, everything changes. On a subconscious level, your mind tells you, "This is great! I don't have that much work to do! I'm free to create!" A clean space actually invites creativity, whereas a messy space invites despair. There is no worse feeling than coming to the office and seeing a huge stack of stuff that has to be done. Your heart sinks. That's why keeping a clean desk helps you create a new standard for yourself, a standard of absolute cleanliness and excellence in everything to do with your workplace. And unless you create for yourself a world-class working environment, you'll find it impossible to operate at a world-class level.

So you've cleared off your desk. Now what about the rest of the office? Your exercise for this chapter is to take your entire team out to the parking lot and walk into your office as a patient would. Take a look around the parking lot. If there are cigarette butts or coffee cups or old newspapers littering the place, it affects the way you are perceived, even if you're not the one responsible for it. If it's a mess, call the landlord. Similarly, are there greasy fingerprints on the glass near your main entrance? Get that cleaned up, too. Do you have old magazines in your reception area? That means old-school dentistry. Get rid of them. Get rid of the pamphlets, too—pamphlets don't sell anything. It's just clutter. If you've got a Visa card sign, get rid of it. That tells your patient that you're all about money and nothing else. Instead, put in educational things that actually help your patients. Don't have signs that do your dirty work like, "Payment is due when services are received." Instead, you should have a system that covers payment, and I would recommend reading *Million Dollar Dentistry* to see how to put one in place.

Keep in mind that people interpret clutter as dirt, and the number one thing they want in a dentist's office is a sterilized area. No desk should have files on top; everything should be stored.

Paint and clean the entire place if it needs it. Take a look up. You might not have noticed that there are dead bugs in your lights or that your ceiling tiles are discolored. Your patient notices those things, especially if you are running behind.

This also means that it's time to reevaluate the tools you use at work. Is your computer a candidate for the PC museum? Is it time to upgrade your telephone or cell phone?

Sometimes people don't know how to de-clutter their offices—what they can keep and what they can toss away. If you're not sure, you can hire an expert in de-cluttering, because there are plenty of people who make a nice living doing for others what they cannot do for themselves: getting the junk out once and for all. However you do it, your standard must be that your office is as meticulously maintained as you now maintain your car.

Okay—let's now leave your immaculate office, jump in your equally immaculate car, and head home. "Uh-oh," I hear you saying. What's that? Your home isn't up to your new standards? Well, it's time to make a transformation there as well. Cast an eye around your home as if you had never been there before. Why are you tolerating those worn-out drapes, the rugs that look as though they came from the Goodwill (or ought to be going there), the scratched-up paneling, the dingy paint? If you look around your house, do you feel as though you've gone to your own yard sale... and overpaid? It's going to take you more than half an hour or forty minutes to get your house in order, but it's time to make a start. Pick one thing in your house that has no particular sentimental value and is too worn-out for words. Throw it in the garbage.

Repeat.

There's really no way to make your home nice until you get rid of the things that make it anything *but* nice. So it's time to give your home an upgrade. Maybe a new coat of paint is necessary. Maybe it's new shutters or French doors. If you were selling the house, you'd drop $10- or $20- or $30,000 on making the place look habitable to the next owner. Aren't you worth it? Isn't it time to spend a few dollars on yourself?

You might be saying, "Gary, I can't afford to drop money into my house!" I'm saying the opposite is true—you can't afford not to. How can you do your best work, how can you be at your most creative, how can you earn the most money…if every night you come home to a place that depresses you? Your home must reflect your values. As George F. Will is often quoted as saying, "We build our buildings, and then they build us." Your home is the place where you spend the most amount of time, although much of it is sleeping. Do you really want to go to sleep at night and wake up in the morning in a place that's beneath your standards? I didn't think so. Take out the trash, pick out a new shade of paint, get the new furniture, spend the money. You and your family are worth it.

In Malcolm Gladwell's book, *The Tipping Point*, he talks about how crime in New York was dramatically reduced, not by adding more policemen, but by boarding up old buildings and cleaning up the environment. Sometimes, cleaning up the environment is all it takes to completely change the climate.

Now let's take a look at the two places in the home that are most representative of your Deserve Level: your closet and your refrigerator. What are you wearing these days? When was the last time you bought yourself nice clothing? Most people's closets are overstocked with items they will never wear again—that is, if they ever even wore them in the first place. In fact, 80 percent of the time, we wear the same 20 percent of our clothing. There must be a whole lot of stuff in your closet you can get rid of because you haven't worn it in the last year. That's generally the rule of thumb that de-clutterers discuss—if you haven't worn something, or used something, within twelve months, it's time for it to go.

Of course, when you empty your closet in this fashion, you often find things that you'd forgotten you had, including articles of clothing you especially liked to wear. How do you know what to keep and what to toss? Again, the standard must be your new, elevated HDL. People with high HDL don't wear old, ratty, tattered clothing. They don't wear it to work and they don't wear it around the house. They don't wear it to the gym and they don't wear it to the store. They always look nice. They care about their appearance, not out of a misplaced sense of egotism or vanity but because they have enough self-respect to demonstrate to the world that they are worthy of having and wearing nice things. There is a Goodwill or other donation center in your neighborhood that would be very grateful for all your castoffs, because those dozens or even hundreds of articles of clothing in your closet that you never wear, and probably never will wear, would be extremely useful to people at lower socioeconomic levels than yourself. What may have little or no value to you has enormous value to others. So you get to help other people at the same time that you help yourself.

Let's talk briefly about your socks and underwear, because, quite frankly, I've seen your sock and underwear drawer, and I'm not impressed! But in all seriousness: another very easy way to measure your HDL is to consider your socks and underwear. This is the stuff that other people seldom see (I'm not here to talk about your social life, so I'll just let that statement stand as it is). Are your socks and underwear religious? By that I mean, are they holy—full of holes? If so, chuck 'em. Nobody wants them…not even people who shop at Goodwill, because their HDLs are higher than that. If you're going to make one investment in your HDL right now, I would have you replace your socks and your undergarments with nice new ones. This is a message that you send to yourself every single day: that you're worthy of nice things. It's tough to be world-class if your underwear isn't.

So now you've cleaned out your car, your workplace, and your home. Let's take a look at what we are accomplishing on a spiritual level. We've already seen that when you create a world-class environment for yourself on the road, at work, and at home, you're sending yourself and others the message that you're world-class. You're setting yourself up to create at the highest level, whether you're creating ideas, money, or love.

On a spiritual level, the act of cleansing your environment in this manner has additional significance. Catherine Ponder, who writes about the spirituality of money, discusses in her books what she calls the "vacuum law of attraction." Ponder writes that nature abhors a vacuum, and when we "create a vacuum" by getting rid of all the extraneous junk and stuff in our lives that we don't need—whether it's old clothes, old carpeting, or a garage full of touch-up paint with colors that we no longer even have in the house—we are actually creating a vacuum or a space. Since nature abhors a vacuum, the universe rushes in to fill the vacuum you've created with even better and nicer things, better experiences, and better relationships.

There's a little bit of pack rat in all of us, but we have to ask why. Why are we hanging onto our college texts? Is it an ego thing, to show the world how smart we are? Do we think we're ever *really* going to reopen any of those textbooks and review the knowledge contained therein? Incidentally, if you graduated more than a month ago, everything in your college textbooks is probably radically out of date. Those things have no particular value anymore, and yet we hang onto them, the way we hang onto so much unnecessary stuff.

It's time to put an end to all of that. Get rid of what you don't need, and that way you'll make room in a physical and spiritual sense for what you do need—better relationships, better things, and a healthier environment for you and the people in your office and your home.

And isn't that what having an elevated HDL is all about?

HDL Highlights

- Every human being lives in a self-created universe, consisting of all the things we use each day to survive, thrive, and better our lives.

- The things in our lives, from the stuff we keep on our desks and in the trunk of our cars to the underwear we wear and the state of our closet, speak volumes about us.

- It's time to put sloppy to bed and create an environment for yourself that demonstrates to you and to the world that you don't just deserve better...you deserve the best.

- A clean space actually invites creativity, whereas a messy space invites despair.

- Create a new standard for yourself: a standard of absolute cleanliness and excellence in everything you do within your workplace. It's time to create for yourself a world-class working environment, because otherwise, you will not operate at a world-class level.

- Get rid of what you don't need, and that way you'll make room in a physical and in a spiritual sense for what you do need—better relationships, better things, and a healthier environment for you and the people in your office and your home.

■ Chapter 7 Exercise / **Freeing Your World**

1. Clean out your car and/or buy a new one.

2. Clear off your desk.

3. Walk your office as if you were a patient, taking note of those things that need to be fixed or altered. Then, make those changes.

4. Do the same at your home.

5. Set realistic deadlines for each.

Grow or Go

ET'S REVIEW WHAT we've accomplished so far. You've recognized that there is a concept called HDL, or Healthy Deserve Level, without which all the self-help seminars, consulting recommendations, and therapy sessions in the world won't mean a thing. You've learned that you've got to identify what you desire in life, which may or may not match up with what others desire for you, or else you run the risk of devoting your life to accomplishing goals that mean little to you or perhaps not accomplishing anything at all. You've also seen that it's vital to replace your internal sense of scarcity, poverty, or lack with prosperity thinking in order to succeed.

In this second part of the book, you have embarked on a massive clean-up process. You've cleaned up your relationship to the past, you've cleaned up your relationship to your word, and in the last chapter, you cleaned up your physical environment, from your car to your workplace to your home. Now we come to the "final frontier" of clean-up necessary in order to maintain your high HDL: the relationships with the people around you.

It's said that our net worth is, plus or minus, the average of the net worths of the five people with whom we have the most contact. It's equally true that your HDL is the average of the HDLs of the five people with whom you spend the most time. So the question becomes: if you are serious about raising your HDL, what do you do if the people in your world aren't serious about raising theirs?

Well, why aren't they? The simple answer is that the human mind is steeped in negativity, and we all tend toward the worst-case scenario much of the time. My definition of an optimist is someone capable of overcoming his or her inherent negativity long enough to hold a positive thought. We all have fear, we all have concern, and, on occasion, we all experience despair and even depression. The problem is that some people latch on to negative thoughts and turn them into movies that they loop endlessly in their minds. They visualize and thus create for themselves the worst-case scenario.

Company may not love misery, but as the expression goes, misery sure loves company. People who are unhappy tend to isolate, but when they do have contact with other people, they often feel the need to pull down the happiness level of those around them. I call this "keeping the tribe alive." Human beings are often tribes of people who feed off each other's misery and unhappiness. When you hear someone say, "I'm so happy for you," don't you get the sense that they really aren't happy, either for you or for themselves?

Why is it that we love building up famous people, only to destroy them at the first possible opportunity? We love to envy others. We love to be jealous. Quite frankly, the more you look at human history, the harder it is to escape the conclusion that we humans love to hate.

Yet, there's no room for envy, jealousy, or hatred on the spiritual plane, and there's no room for these emotions in individuals seeking to raise their HDL. So the question we now have to ask ourselves is: what do you do about the people in your life who do not have a high HDL? The simple answer is that they must grow...or go.

The starting point is not to criticize or condemn them for their low HDL. After all, you chose to have them in your life, if you are over the age of eighteen. These are the people with whom you are in a relationship, whether it's a working or a social one. It's a free country, and as the expression goes, among adults there are no victims, only volunteers. In other words, if the people in your life have a low HDL, you volunteered to hang around them, to get into a relationship with them, to work with them, to work for them, to have them as patients, or to keep them around in some form or fashion. It makes sense that you did, because until not all that long ago, your HDL was as low as theirs!

The difference between you and them is that you have read and presumably acted upon the suggestions in the first seven chapters of this book. As a result, your HDL is soaring, which may make you something of a curiosity or even a source of upset to those around you. Maybe they feel threatened by the fact that you are taking more seriously than ever the concepts of integrity. Maybe they feel envious of you for keeping your word. Maybe they don't want a clean car!

I love the quote, "All people always do the best they can with the awareness they have. You can only expand a person's awareness with his or her permission." They are doing the best with what they've got. You're the one who has suddenly started to clean up your act, your desk, and your office. You've gone from bringing home Häagen-Dazs to bringing home carrots and cucumbers. In fact, while you're casting a critical eye on the low HDL of the people in your world, they're probably looking at you and thinking, "You're no fun anymore!"

That's certainly not the point of having a high HDL. In fact, high HDL people have the most fun of anyone. But it kind of reminds me of the story about the guy who decided that he was going to transform his whole life. So he goes to the gym, works out, eats right, gets a great new body, buys a beautiful new wardrobe, goes to the tanning booth—the whole nine yards. When all is said and done, he looks fantastic. The very day he makes his goal weight, he steps off the curb in his fantastic new clothes...and gets run over by a Mac truck.

He goes to heaven.

He meets God. He says, "God, how could you do this to me?"

And God replies, "To be honest, I didn't recognize you."

The people in your life may not recognize the new you! That's okay. Give them some time to get used to your new standards. Developing a high HDL is not an excuse to become smug or holier than thou, however. Incidentally, this is the way human beings were meant to live, so it's not appropriate to take credit for something that you should have been doing all along. Keeping your word? Not eating like a pig? Wearing underwear without any holes in it? For this, you want a medal? I don't think so!

The serious point is that you have begun to live life on a different plane from those around you, and people often feel threatened or disconnected when those in their world make meaningful changes. You might think, for example, that when a co-worker makes a dramatic lifestyle change toward better health, when she starts exercising regularly, eating right, and shedding those extra pounds, that everyone in the office will rejoice. The reality is often quite the opposite. The other people in the office may feel threatened by the change. Maybe they don't want to look at their own eating patterns. Perhaps they will feel less-than or threatened, and their instinctual urge to compete and dominate will kick in. Instead of demonstrating support and happiness for that person, they withdraw or retreat. Change, even positive change, threatens things.

Psychologists often speak of the family unit as a mobile. Touch one element of it and the entire things quivers. The same is true in the workplace or in any situation where individuals have frequent interactions. So it's your responsibility not to judge or condemn others for being the way you were not all that long ago. At the same time, you have a responsibility to yourself, and to them, to investigate whether it might be possible for these individuals to join you on your new, higher HDL.

It's a little like speaking a new language—the language

of the soul, if you will. Everyone else in your family is still speaking English, and here you come, speaking the Soul Language. Unless subtitles are magically appearing on your chest like in a foreign film, the other people in your life may have a hard time understanding what you're trying to say. So it's important to have conversations with the most influential people in your life, discuss with them what you are doing, and determine whether you and they can find common ground.

As an exercise, I'd like to suggest that you take a few moments to make a list of the ten or twenty people in your life with whom you have the most contact, the people who influence your moods and behavior the most on a day-to-day basis. If you're married or in a relationship, your partner or spouse would head the list. Then come your children, if you have any, followed by your parents, especially if you live with them or are in frequent or close contact with them. Even if you're not in regular contact with your parents, the way they think probably still has a powerful influence on the way *you* think. As the expression goes, "Our parents know how to press our buttons. After all, they installed them."

Next, look to the workplace. With whom do you interact in the office on a regular basis? Who are the key team members in your working life right now? They may be people who work for you, or maybe they are vendors or colleagues. Who goes on your list from work?

Next, consider your friends. Who do you call, e-mail, IM, or text when you have a free moment? Who do you hang with? Who do you play golf with? Who's your walking partner? Who's your gym buddy? They go on the list, too.

Finally, who advises you? Are you in regular contact with a therapist, coach, consultant, financial advisor, accountant, or attorney? Who's on your team? If you're in regular contact with such individuals, and they have regular contact or influence in your life, put them down on the list.

Now take a look at your list and ask yourself what you notice about the HDLs of these people. Chances are, they're all bunched up, pretty much in the same place—the same place where you were until you began to identify the importance of HDL in your own life. Frankly, it's rare that people who have very high HDLs hang out with people who don't. High HDL people, as I've mentioned throughout this book, enjoy life more than low HDL people. They often have more money, and even if they have the same amount of money as someone else, they simply have more fun spending it, investing it, or using it in worthy ways. It's not just about money, however. It's really got to do with where you and those around you have your focus and attention.

It's been my experience—and I've seen this described again and again in books—that the higher up you go in any organization, the nicer the people are. This flies in the face of what most people think about powerful individuals. For the most part, in the public mind, the most successful individuals are the hard-driving, egotistical types—the Jack Welches or Donald Trumps of the world. But in reality, successful people are often the nicest people. Ironically, in a world that everybody thinks is dog eat dog, these people have never eaten anything more canine-like than a hot dog! They understand that the world isn't like college, where whoever gets the best grades wins. Instead, they understand that the world is like high school—the people who are the most likable, the team players, the people who go out for Key Club, the people who make the yearbook happen... *those* are the ones who have the best time and generally go on to the greatest level of success. It's a people world, and everything that's good in life comes to us through people. So generally, the most successful people, the ones with the highest HDLs, are also the individuals who get the most out of life...and give the most back.

So what about your HDL partners? I use the word partners intentionally, because they are partners with you in co-creating your HDL. If you are surrounded by low HDL people, it's hard to maintain a positive outlook. If you are among people who like to complain, it's hard to see the good in people. It's easy to fall into their pattern of complaint and criticism, instead of recognizing that there are all kinds of people in the world, and not all of them are worthy of our criticism. Indeed, if there was one trait that separated low HDL people from high HDL people, it would be the tendency to criticize or complain about others.

How else can you identify the HDLs of the people around you? Well, put them to the tests to which you've subjected yourself over the course of this book. Do they keep their word? If they say they're going to do something or be somewhere, is it so? Can you count on them in matters large and small? What do their possessions, furnishings, workplaces, home spaces, wardrobes, and diet tell you about them? Do you get the sense that they are coming from abundance, or are they coming from lack? Do they know what they want in life? Are they going for it? Do they have that combination of relishing life and the "divine dissatisfaction" that pushes people to develop themselves to the max? Do they live in the present with an eye on a big future, or are they stuck in the past? We've all got blind spots—it's impossible for any of us to have complete, 100 percent objectivity about our own lives. But are the blind spots of the people around you so big that they create tunnel vision, where all they can see is what's negative in themselves, in others, and in the world?

I think you're catching my drift. These people might have been ideal for you back when your HDL was low. But now that you have taken on a commitment to becoming the highest and best version of yourself possible, are you surrounding yourself with others who do likewise?

This is not the time to go on a crusade to get other people to follow your lead, clean out their closets, get the Taco Bell wrappers out of the back seat of their cars, and buy new socks. This is the time to ask yourself whether the relationships that are the most dominant in your life will continue to work for you, now that you have jettisoned your low HDL and taken on an entirely new stance toward what your life can be. Essentially, we're not asking people to change their lives, because we don't have a right to do that. Instead, we do have a right—and furthermore, a responsibility to ourselves—to consider the way their words, behaviors, attitudes, and outlooks affect us. And we do get to have conversations with these individuals, much like I did with my grandmother, where we ask them to modify an aspect of their behavior that no longer works in our relationship with them.

For example, let's say that there's someone on your team who tends to complain a lot. You might not have ever seen the problem that complaining causes or the negative energy that it creates. But now you do. You have a right to say, "Look. I really enjoy my relationship with you, but I just don't want to listen to any more complaining. Would it be possible for us to have conversations that include you sharing what you have to say with a solution, not just a problem?"

It's all about delivering a straight message. You can tell your friend, partner, spouse, co-worker, client, or customer your truth…one time. If they get it, great. If they don't get it, you've got to get that they don't get it! We cannot harp on this message. We can deliver it once, lovingly and courteously, and then we have to step back and see what the results are. It's unhealthy, unnecessary, and essentially pointless to create a dynamic with another person in which we're always right and we're always making them wrong. That's not what a high HDL is all about.

What we want to do is transform the relationship so that both individuals in it are coming from high HDL, instead of negativity and criticism.

A funny thing happened as I was writing these words. The phone in my office rang and my colleague took the call. It turned out to be a former client who, shall we say, does not place integrity among his top three values. Am I being delicate enough? There's a reason he's a *former* client! He's a person with whom I found it impossible to create a positive relationship.

In cases like that, the only appropriate relationship…is no relationship at all. The problem is that this isn't always possible, because the person with the lowest HDL on your list may be your partner, your spouse, or the patient you think you can't afford to lose. The simple fact is that you will not always be able to create the kind of high HDL relationships with everyone in your world that you might wish. What typically happens, though, is that over time, the low HDL people in your life fade away. They de-select themselves…as long as you continue to take the high HDL road.

Not all relationships are meant to last forever. The ones that are inappropriate for you as your HDL rises will diminish in importance over time. When they go away, it will have the same effect in your life as when you created a vacuum in your wardrobe closet, in your kitchen pantry, and in your workspace. You'll be creating a vacuum that the universe will rush in to fill with better-quality relationships, and those relationships will be with individuals whose HDLs match your new, higher one. I don't believe couples break up over religious, ethnic, racial, philosophical, or political differences. I do believe that marriages and relationships break up when one person has a consistently higher HDL than the other. This is a topic that could and probably should be discussed in a coaching or therapy setting, especially if there are children involved.

The main thing is this: The people surrounding you in your life have enormous impact on your HDL. Just as you became more comfortable with your past, grew in terms of integrity, and cleaned up your physical environment, it is equally important to review the key relationships in your life. Ask yourself: are these individuals helping me grow my HDL, or are they holding me back? In most cases, the message that you will end up delivering, through words or actions, to those around you with low HDL is: grow or go. You simply cannot afford to have relationships past their expiration dates holding you back from becoming the person you are meant to be.

In the first section of this book, we discussed seeing what HDL is all about. In this section, we've worked on freeing our ability to have that high HDL. In the final section, we will discuss the question of "being" a high HDL individual. What does it mean to live an impeccable, world-class, high HDL life? Join me in the final section of this book, and we'll take that journey together.

HDL Highlights

- It's said that our net worth is, plus or minus, the average of the net worths of the five people with whom we have the most contact. It's equally true that your HDL is the average of the HDLs of the five people with whom you spend the most time.

- It's important to have conversations with the most influential people in your life, discuss with them what you are doing, and determine whether you and they can find common ground.

- Generally, the most successful people, the ones with the highest HDLs, are also the individuals who get the most out of life...and give the most back.

- If you are surrounded by negative people, it's hard to maintain a positive outlook.

- Just as you became more comfortable with your past, grew in terms of integrity, and cleaned up your physical environment, it is equally important to review the key relationships in your life. Ask yourself: are these individuals helping you grow your HDL, or are they holding you back? If they're holding you back, your message to them should be simple: either grow, or go.

■ Chapter 8 Exercise / **Grow or Go**

Take a blank sheet of paper and put yourself in the center. Write on each corner: Social, Work, Family, and Other. List the names of all the important people in each of these departments of your life. What conversations do you need to have with each of these people? Keep it all on one page, so that you can see it.

Become an HDL leader—start pioneering a movement in your world to raise the HDL of those around you. Prioritize among the people you know. In other words, only bring this idea to those who are most open and willing. There are always pioneers, frontiersmen, and settlers. You're a pioneer, so stick to your own on this one. Not everyone will be an early adapter, either on your team or among your patients. But let the vital conversation about HDL begin. Look and listen for your team members and significant others to make changes that are congruent with a high HDL person. Then, stand back and watch as the HDL in your personal sphere of influence continues to grow and flourish…all thanks to you.

Part III

BEING IT / *The Payoff You'll Love*

Chapter 9

UBU, UBC, and CBC

HOLLYWOOD CAN SPEND $250 million or more
creating a blockbuster movie. But how do they get *you*
to want to see it?

In the movie industry, they understand that it takes
at least five "impressions" on potential moviegoers before
they are ready to plunk down their hard-earned dollars on
any one particular film. The movie might offer the greatest
stars on the planet, the most exciting story, and the greatest
special effects...but until moviegoers are reminded about
the film an average of five different times, they won't stop
and say, "I've got to see it."

Impressions include an ad you see on a billboard while
you're driving, an ad on the side of a city bus, a banner
ad on a Web site you visit, an interview with one of the
stars that you see on TV, an article in a newspaper or magazine about the making of the film, a radio contest to win
free tickets to the opening in your town, and so on. Put
it all together and, once you've got those five impressions,

something clicks inside you and you make a mental note to go see that film.

In dentistry, this is what I call the five times trust transfer. Essentially, the patient needs to hear and see the problem, consequence, and solution associated with his or her condition five times before they are sold on the recommended treatment plan. The five impressions include interactions between the hygienist and the patient, the hygienist and the dentist, the dentist and the patient, the hygienist and the treatment coordinator, and the treatment coordinator and the patient. When this happens, the patient will have confidence in the solution and will buy the treatment plan.

It's not all that different with developing a high HDL. I don't want to give the impression that if you follow the cookie-cutter recipe, you'll get there in an instant and never look back. That's not how human nature works. Pretty much everything important in life involves taking three steps forward and one step back. So just as the movie industry and dental practice require five impressions before you or your patients are ready to commit, so it is with HDL. It takes multiple steps, multiple efforts, multiple commitments to get where you want to go. And that's okay, because if you stick around long enough and hang with the process, eventually you'll find the concept of living with high HDL becoming more and more familiar.

The following metaphor helps illustrate my point. Imagine a group of firemen who rush into a burning tenement, only to find that the panicked residents are not speaking English. Instead, the residents are trying to communicate with the firemen in their native languages, because in crisis, we always go back to our first language. In the same way, when the first moment of challenge to your new, high HDL comes along, it's not likely that you're going to respond in a totally HDL manner. If you're like most people, you'll find yourself instinctively speaking your "first" language—the response process of a person whose HDL isn't as high as yours has become. That person isn't you any longer.

The process of moving from low HDL to high HDL begins when we take the steps that I've outlined in the first two sections of this book. But we're dealing with human nature, which tends to be rooted in the past and takes a little while before it catches up with changes in programming. You really are reprogramming your entire mind to respond to situations in entirely new ways, and to create new worlds of success and happiness for yourself and those around you. No wonder it's not an overnight process! So if you find yourself backsliding, if you find yourself shouting in your native language in a moment of crisis, don't take that as a sign of failure or a low HDL. Just accept the fact that it took you years to develop the thinking patterns that governed your life…right up until the moment you and I started working together. All those years of thinking aren't going to be undone in a single moment.

It reminds me of a *Peanuts* cartoon I saw when I was growing up. Lucy was going around telling Linus all kinds of ridiculous things like, "The rain starts from the ground and goes up into the sky, and then it turns around and comes back and gets everything wet." Or, "Grass grows down, not up." The punch line was Charlie Brown looking sadly at the reader and saying, "Poor Linus. He's going to have to spend twelve more years than everyone else in school, just unlearning everything Lucy taught him."

It's not going to take you twelve years to unlearn everything you learned about life. But it will take more than twelve seconds or twelve minutes. Just as Hollywood requires five impressions to get you to make a decision, it's going to take multiple instances of "HDL moment" situations requiring the application of high HDL in order to get the results you want— in other words, before you're totally onboard with this new approach to life.

The transition might seem tricky, and it might even seem challenging. Remember, it's about progress. If you notice a moment or instance where the level of your HDL is challenged, step back and reflect with gratitude. This marks progress. Then, keep going. Before long, operating from high HDL will be second nature. But you do have to go through three distinctive phases first.

I divide these three phases into groupings that I call UBU, UBC, and CBC. These funny little acronyms actually stand for very important concepts. UBU means "uncomfortable being uncomfortable." UBC means "uncomfortable being comfortable." CBC means "comfortable being comfortable." These are the three phases of HDL growth through which each of us must pass.

Let's take a look at each of them in turn.

In the UBU phase, nothing seems to fit right. A situation arises at home, at work, or in some other department of our lives, and the natural instinct is to revert to our old tendencies—to be the immigrant in the burning tenement shouting in his or her native tongue. That's okay. Indeed, that's to be expected and even encouraged. It would be foolhardy to expect that any of us could toss away a lifetime of behavioral traits in an instant. Again, that's just not how human nature works.

In my experience working with dental teams, it takes not just the five experiences that Hollywood requires, but as many as twenty separate HDL moments before a person moves out of the UBU stage. A stimulus arises, and the natural tendency of a person in that moment might be to complain. Or to overeat. Or to practice inappropriate behavior within a relationship. Or to cheat or fudge on something at work. It's going to take as many as twenty different such moments before the new high HDL approach to life kicks in automatically. There's going to be discomfort in that process, and there's also going to be impatience. That's because most of us don't just want what we want—we want it now. As Carrie Fisher wrote in *Postcards From the Edge*, "The problem with immediate gratification is that it takes too long." So that's why I call this stage the UBU stage, because most people are uncomfortable making the shift to high HDL…and they're uncomfortable *being* uncomfortable. They tend to experience high levels of impatience, anger, and frustration during this phase.

Most people think of frustration as a negative emotion. Not me. I see it as entirely positive and healthy. It means that you are no longer willing to tolerate the way things were, or more importantly, the way *you* were. It means that the old rules about how you handled situations, challenges, and crises are no longer acceptable to you, even if you find yourself falling back into your old ways of thinking, speaking, and behaving. In the UBU phase, we find ourselves uncomfortable being uncomfortable because of our desire to be at a higher level overnight. We can commit to change in an instant, but to live the change takes a little bit longer. And that's a good thing.

Most of us are impatient once we see what we truly want. So if you're feeling uncomfortable, if you're feeling impatient, if you're feeling frustrated, and even if you're feeling angry at yourself, it's okay. I understand! You are going through the first stage of HDL growth, and this stage simply can't be skipped.

It's been said that the two greatest tragedies in life are individuals trying to skip a phase of their development, and individuals who stay stuck in a particular phase of their development. HDL is a stern taskmaster—it requires us to repeat lessons over and over again until we finally break through. When the student is ready, the teacher shows up. Until the student is ready, challenges will reappear. So if you're feeling uncomfortable in the first stage of HDL growth, the UBU stage, that's really exactly where you're supposed to be. It's not a punishment for the way you lived your life in the past. It's simply the awareness of the disconnect between the way you lived and the way you desire to live now.

Back to Hollywood. You've seen those five impressions and you say to your spouse, partner, boyfriend, girlfriend, or just to yourself, "I want to go see that movie." And you do. You made the decision, and you're ready to act. You're now in stage two. In HDL terms, I call stage two the UBC phase, because now you have moved to a place where you are uncomfortable being comfortable. In other words, when an HDL moment kicks in at home, work, or anywhere else, you have now ingrained new behavioral, thinking, and speaking traits. You don't respond the way you did in the past, in that instinctive and perhaps negative manner. A situation arises and whereas before you might have complained, you find yourself biting your tongue. You've just finished a cup of coffee in your car, and instead of tossing it into the back seat, you put the cup carefully back in the bag so that it doesn't spill and stain your car's upholstery. A situation at the office arises, and suddenly you find yourself handling it in a new way—you return the patient's phone call despite the fear you feel. Or you tell your team that a particular project isn't going to work and you stand your ground in that difficult conversation.

By now, your behavior reflects your "new and improved" HDL, but your mindset still isn't quite with the program. You say to yourself things like, "Wow, where did those words come from?" Or, "What made me act that way? I didn't know I had it in me!" In other words, the HDL moment arrives and you're doing things the way you want to do them, instead of the way you handled them in the past. Yet there's still a level of discomfort, because you almost don't recognize yourself!

Once you reach the level of UBC, shifts happen in your relationships at home, at work, and everywhere else. Now it's no longer just about how you feel. Your team begins to step up their game and come from a place of higher HDL as well. Or they begin to disappear out of your life. In my experience, once people start expressing themselves and generally behaving in a higher HDL manner, as we discussed in the UBU phase, other people start to sit up and take notice. Maybe you've had to speak politely to one of your hygienists and ask her to stop complaining about your team leader. Or maybe you've had a conversation with your spouse, partner, boyfriend, or girlfriend in which you've expressed a desire that in the past you haven't been able to put into words. In other words, your environment is changing because you've drawn that HDL line in the sand.

During the UBC phase, whenever there's a low HDL moment in your life involving some important person at work or home, there's a high probability that both you and the other person are uncomfortable. That's because, for whatever reason, the exchange is not living up to the high HDL standards that you have imposed on your world. To put it bluntly: discomfort is guaranteed during this phase. But when you think about it, it makes sense. You have set new terms for your life, and in so doing, you have set new terms for your relationships. It's now up to other people to take on your new standards.

The exciting thing is that for the most part, people want to do so. They want to live their lives in a manner congruent with high HDL.

By and large, people want to keep their word. They want to tell the truth. They want to feel good about themselves. And now here you come, Mr. or Ms. High HDL, making everybody around you elevate their game. Are they all going to thank you for this? Absolutely not! A lot of people would choose comfort over excellence any day, and you are forcing everyone in your world to step out of their comfort zones and excel. Not everyone's going to thank you for it. So don't be surprised if there will be a little bit of pushback or blow-back from the people in your world who think that it's all fine and dandy for you to step up and have a different life…but they sure as heck don't want to be dragged along with you. If they don't like it, they're just going to have to adjust, aren't they?

Now you understand why I call this second phase of HDL growth UBC, or uncomfortable being comfortable. The comfort comes from the fact that it now takes you much less effort to achieve the kind of positive HDL moments and results that might have come as a bit of a struggle during the first uncomfortable being uncomfortable stage. So you're starting to reap the rewards, and you're starting to see that this thing really works. The discomfort comes because it's new, it's still a little strange, and it involves other people—not all of whom will be as intrigued by the possibility of personal growth as you are.

If there's one tool that comes into play the most during the UBC phase, it's the ability to come face-to-face with things and people. It now becomes radically easier to have open and honest communication about any situations that are not world-class. In one of our offices in Kansas, they call such moments "Mountain Dew moments," because at one point, one of their team members sat the doctor down and said, "Dr. Jeff, I need to have a Mountain Dew with you and talk something over." She was concerned that he wasn't living up to one of his agreements, and she turned out to be right! So ever since, in their office, if someone says, "I need to have a Mountain Dew moment with you," they all know what that means. It means that they are about to sit down and have a conversation to confront something that isn't entirely world-class.

The challenge for most people is that confrontation is really, really hard. It's uncomfortable. It's easier to just go with the status quo than to make things better. You know all the expressions—the devil you know is better than the devil you don't, that sort of thing. So it's time to let go of those old tapes that say you are not permitted to have polite confrontations with people, and instead recognize that if you're going to be world-class, you've got to be willing to sit down with people and have a Mountain Dew with them in order to talk things out.

During the UBC phase, we don't do things perfectly. Sometimes we are aching to backslide; to do things the way we used to do them; to go back to our old methods, approaches, and strategies. While we don't have to do so, the tendency is still going to be there. That's why the emotion that predominates during the second phase is uncertainty—the understanding that we aren't going to get it perfectly every time, that we're going to have the desire to backslide, and that HDL, while it's magnificent, isn't the magic bullet that transforms our lives in an instant.

Another emotion associated with this second phase is resignation, where you tell yourself, "I'm *never* going to get this." Yeah, you are! It might take you a little longer than you thought, because again, we don't get instant high HDL the way we want it the very first second we start thinking about it. It takes time to create. It takes time to adjust to your new way of looking at yourself, others, and the world. So if you start telling yourself things like "I can't do this" or "It's never going to work," or if you're trying to institute high HDL in your home or your workplace and you start saying to yourself, "We'll never get this," or, "It's never going to work here," take heart. That's exactly the emotion that people feel at this stage of the process. If anything, use that sense of resignation as a signal to yourself that you are on track, that you are going where you're supposed to be going, and that things are headed in the right direction. It sounds crazy, but that's really how HDL works.

This is also the phase where it is up to you to become more responsible. I don't mean responsible in terms of declaring things are right or wrong, good or bad. I'm talking about being responsible as a cause, as the cause of things. It's about making a move from saying "What just happened?" to making things happen. We are either causes or effects in life. People with low HDL tend to be at the mercy of situations, people, and things. Their cars are always breaking down, and always at the worst possible time. They run out of gas on the highway. There's nothing in the cupboard for dinner. Things just don't go their way. That's no way to live, and that's why you've made the move from a low medium HDL existence to a world-class, high HDL way of life. So now is the time to recognize that blaming, criticizing, condemning, and making other people wrong is no longer compatible with your impeccable existence. If you feel uncomfortable when the urge to criticize, condemn, or complain arises within you, that's good. It means that you're recognizing that you no longer want to live in that fashion. You want to bring unwavering commitment to this new way of life.

Typically, when things go well for dentists with low HDL, they self-sabotage. They keep themselves on a roller coaster of success and failure, never quite comfortable with success, but never comfortable enough with failure to admit complete defeat. They exhaust themselves on two treadmills—a treadmill of being busy and a treadmill of hiring consultants. I call this consultant fatigue. So often, dentists bring people in to get a different result, but they haven't expanded their Deserve Level. As a result, they procrastinate, because at their core they don't believe they can expand and accomplish what they set out to accomplish. When they bring someone in, they don't follow through. The fear is that they will succeed, thus invalidating their low Deserve Level with which they are so comfortable.

Raising your HDL kills this dreaded consultant fatigue by inviting world-class expansion, and thereby providing sustained results. If you're like most of the dentists I consult, you want a solution so badly…but you haven't even considered that changing your Deserve Level might be the very solution you so desperately seek. You possess the solution. You *are* the solution. Just as the lion in the *Wizard of Oz* already had the courage, the tin man a brain, and the scarecrow a heart, everything you need is already inside you.

Back to the treadmill. Break free from it. If not, it can be like building on quicksand—the quicksand of low HDL that takes people and their success down, down, down. In the first phase of HDL growth, UBU, or uncomfortable being uncomfortable, there's a tendency to revert to that roller coaster mentality. In the second phase, where we are uncomfortable being comfortable, we still might go for one or two or even ten or twelve more roller coaster rides, but they're usually shorter and less exciting (and I mean exciting in a bad way). The good news is that this level of comfort within discomfort eventually subsides and instead turns into something even better—much better, in fact. That's the level I call CBC, or "comfortable being comfortable."

This is the place where you're really in a groove with your high HDL life processes and habits. In a crisis or confrontation, you take the high road, making full use of your world-class, high HDL attitude. The thoughts that you think and the words that come out of your mouth reflect that high HDL. You create, and then you are able to enjoy the fruits of your creation…so you keep on creating more. You're building on a solid emotional, spiritual, and physical foundation instead of building on quicksand. Every time you get to a new level, you see that there is another level beyond that. You desire to reach that new level—not because you're on an insatiable treadmill of accomplishment like you were in the past, and not because you're on that roller coaster of success and defeat that's always defined you. Instead, you want to create simply for the joy and beauty of creation, for the ability to serve others, and to maximize your enjoyment of your own life. You never have to worry about becoming bored when you are comfortable being comfortable. You never reach that "Is that all there is?" phase of life that so many successful people encounter.

The analogy I like to use is that you've made the decision to try every restaurant in New York City. It takes years, and by the time you finish, you've got to start all over again, because thousands of new restaurants have opened up in the meantime. I've heard people use other analogies to describe this process—painting the Golden Gate Bridge, for example, or painting the White House, because as soon as the workers finish the job, they have to start all over. But that particular example doesn't sound very appealing to me. Personally, I'd rather try every restaurant in New York! Wouldn't you?

When you're comfortable being comfortable, there's an abundance of new experiences awaiting you. Now you're in a place where you are responsible, unwavering, and unattached to results. You've surrendered your need to control outcomes, which means you actually get better outcomes than ever before. Many people allow themselves what I call linear growth—their income improves by a few percentage points, their relationships get a tiny bit better, and their physical well-being improves marginally. But what about exponential growth? This is what's available to you in every facet of your life once you reach the CBC phase.

Once you've made it to the comfortable being comfortable phase, the people around you are deeply affected by your new strength as well. You'll find yourself elevating their game without even intending to do so. There are fewer and fewer "Mountain Dew moments" with those in your immediate world, because they understand that you play by world-class rules now, and so must they. By and large, they will. Things just keep spiraling upward, instead of coasting downward. You don't feel guilty about your success.

I want to take a moment to say that there's an important distinction between investing in yourself and filling up that I.V. like we talked about in Chapter Four. When you invest in yourself during the CBC phase, your HDL automatically goes up. I'm talking about having the nice car, the nice ward-robe, the nice home—all the nice accouterments of life. But if you're getting things simply because the brand name will impress other people, forget it. That's back to shooting up with your I.V. I'm talking about getting nice things—the things that demonstrate a high sense of self-regard. Overspending leads to an image of frivolity; spending lovingly and even on occasion lavishly on oneself indicates high HDL. The more you spend on yourself, the more money will come to you.

Many people misconstrue HDL and think it's all about arrogance, greed, and materialism. In reality, it's the opposite of that—it's an entirely different concept. Suddenly you are on a plane where material things come to you, money comes to you, love comes to you, success at work comes to you, and your dreams come to you, easily and quickly. It's as though you've found Aladdin's Lamp. All you have to do is just simply give it away and allow it to come back. This is what I call the law of reciprocity. If you want more love, love more. If you want more respect, respect others more. The more you put out to the world, the more you will get back.

We often confuse spirituality with asceticism. We think that if we aren't a monk sitting on top of a hill, contemplating our breath, we aren't spiritual. I'm here to say that you can be just as spiritual as that monk while you are sitting behind the wheel of your brand new BMW 7 Series, at your desk at work, going over your investments, or being with your loved ones. I'm talking about an "in-the-world spirituality." The good news is that if you feel compelled to go off and sit on a hilltop somewhere, you can now afford to do so. The *bad* news is that last time I checked, just about every hilltop worth sitting on belongs to someone, and they'll want to charge you rent!

Now let's look at CBC, or comfortable being comfortable, in terms of effort and result. In the first phase, UBU, uncomfortable being uncomfortable, it might have taken twenty units of energy to create one unit of result. By the time you got to UBC, or the second phase of uncomfortable being comfortable, you probably reached a state of parity between effort and outcome. Now, in CBC, or comfortable being comfortable, one unit of effort produces twenty units of result.

It's a beautiful way to live life, isn't it? It's couldn't be farther removed from the fear-based approach to money, success, love, health, fitness, and spirituality that defines most of our lives. In the CBC phase, as Fred Astaire used to say, you are no longer dancing. Instead, you *are* the dance; you *are* the music. You are an extension of the world's spirituality instead of a person who is fighting against it. In sports terms, you're letting the game come to you. You're like a Wayne Gretzky, skating to where the puck will be so that you can have an easy score.

When you reach this level of consciousness and awareness, you experience ease, freedom, and connection to people around you so that you're able to give them exactly what they need when they need it. At the same time you're giving yourself what you need, even before you know you want it. The game is coming to you. Is this a reasonable expectation? Not in normal, everyday terms. But for people who have high HDLs, this is entirely reasonable. I love the quote from George Bernard Shaw about the fact that unreasonable individuals are the people who make things happen in life. Is it reasonable to have such unreasonable expectations? Yes, absolutely. When your HDL is high enough, there are no limits on you. No financial limits. No relationship limits. No production or collection limits. The only boundaries on you are the choices you make with regard to your own morality and integrity. You've learned to keep your word to the universe, and now the universe begins to unload its storehouse of treasures on you.

So those are the three phases of HDL. We moved from uncomfortable being uncomfortable, to uncomfortable being comfortable, and finally, to comfortable being comfortable. Once you've made your way to CBC, there's only one thing left: learning how to stay there.

HDL Highlights:

- When you set your sights on achieving a high HDL as a state of being, you really are reprogramming your entire mind to respond to situations in entirely new ways, and to create new worlds of success and happiness for yourself and those around you.

- If you find yourself backsliding, if you find yourself shouting in your native language in a moment of crisis, don't take that as a sign of failure or a low HDL. Instead, look at it as a learning process—a necessary step on the path to changing the way you live your life.

- UBU means "uncomfortable being uncomfortable." UBC means "uncomfortable being comfortable." CBC means "comfortable being comfortable." These are the three phases of HDL growth through which each of us must pass.

- It's going to take as many as twenty different UBU moments before the new high HDL approach to life kicks in automatically.

- Once you reach the level of UBC, shifts happen in your relationships at home, at work, and everywhere else.

- When you're comfortable being comfortable (CBC), there's an abundance of new experiences awaiting you. Now you're in a place where you are responsible, unwavering, and unattached to results. You've surrendered your need to control outcomes, which means you actually get better outcomes than ever before.

- Remember my *Wizard of Oz* analogy. The solution you are seeking exists within yourself. Embrace yourself and welcome a higher HDL…the HDL you've deserved all along.

■ Chapter 9 Exercise / **UBU, UBC, and CBC**

Create an "and" game instead of an "or" game for yourself. What would happen if you had all the time *and* money in the world? What would you be, do, and have? Life is no longer about deciding between things; it's not a choice of one thing or the other. You can have both. So use the word "and" as opposed to "or."

One of my clients in Kansas is creating a community center for teens *and* is the top dentist in his town. A Las Vegas client is creating a dog rescue center *and* has a world-class practice. An Ohio dentist and his partner have a LEED-certified eco-dental office, because being green means the world to them—*and* they're on target for $5 million this year. Still another client renovated his office to make it virtually indistinguishable from a Hard Rock Café. He's the Hard Rock Dentist!

Who are you? What do you want your office to say about you? This is an opportunity for you to attract patients of similar mind.

What do you want your office to reflect? Envision it. Clip pictures that match your visions. Create a vision board with your team and invite them to participate and provide their visions, too. Collage. Brainstorm. Create your ideal team vision on a board in your team room. Then, once your dreams are all but ready to leap off the page…go get 'em!

Keeping on Track

ARLY ON IN THIS BOOK, we discussed the image of the race car driver continuing to spin around the track long after he received the checkered flag, totally unaware that he had already won. The other drivers had gone home, the stands had emptied, the grounds crew was picking up the trash from the stands, and yet our lone racer was still out there spinning, acting as if the race was still on when he should have been at home celebrating.

By now, you've learned that having a high HDL is the key to happiness, joy, and freedom. When your HDL is high, you recognize how victorious you are in life, how much you have created for yourself, and how much you have created for others. It's not enough to win—you have to know, in your heart, that you've won. Imagine if the driver who won the Daytona 500 stepped out of his racing car and turned down the trophy, the million dollar prize money, the accolades from the fans, and the kiss from his joyous wife. You'd feel bad for a guy like that, wouldn't you? Well, most of us have been that guy at one time or another—unwilling to recognize that we deserved the fruits of victory, and unable to experience the sweetness of life, despite the outward trappings we may possess.

If you've read this far, then you now know the real secret of life—that you get in life not just what you think about, or negotiate for, or "put out into the universe," but what you think you deserve. Now you know how to raise your Deserve Level to the point where it's healthy enough that you can accept that trophy, that million dollar check, that applause, and that love. It's now a part of you.

So our discussion moves from the question of what a Healthy Deserve Level is and how to create it to an equally intriguing and important question: how to sustain it. Today, sustainability is one of the most important terms when it comes to the environment, agriculture, and the way we live our lives. We want to create a sustainable future for ourselves, for those around us, and for the generations that follow us. We recognize that if we don't create a sustainable future, we will not continue to enjoy the blessings that our physical world provides.

It's no different with HDL and dentistry. It's not just about creating a high HDL—it's about creating *sustainable* systems and processes. So in this chapter, I'd like to share with you some highly successful approaches to structures and accountability to keep yourself on track and make your high HDL truly sustainable.

The first distinction I want to share with you is that you are no longer trying to *get* somewhere. You're already there! Now it's about *being* the person with that high HDL...not just for a day or a week or a month, but for the rest of your life.

Studies have shown that after two weeks, we retain only 10 percent of the information we've read in a particular book...unless we act on that information. What does it mean to act on information? The first thing we can do is talk it through to ourselves. If someone asked you what high HDL meant, what would you tell them? If you can put in your own words what I've sought to share with you in this book, you will double your retention of the ideas you've discovered here.

Doubling something sounds great, but let's not get too excited. After all, we're just going from 10 percent retention to 20 percent retention. That's really not good enough for a sustainable high HDL. Let me put it this way: of all the ideas you've read in this book so far, which ideas would you be willing to forget 80 or 90 percent of for the rest of your life?

If you have found this concept of HDL (and my strategy for creating it) compelling enough to read this far, first I want to thank you. That's a great sign of respect that you've paid me, to devote your time to these thoughts. So I want to honor you for that. But more importantly, I want you to be able to use these ideas for the rest of your life. So doubling a retention rate from 10 to 20 percent still means that 80 percent of the material in this book won't be in your future. That just won't cut it—not if you truly are committed to being world-class.

That's why I want to suggest that you find yourself an accountability partner for HDL. An accountability partner is simply someone to whom you explain the concept of HDL and whom you ask to help keep you on track. It's all but impossible for individuals to be objective about their own situations. When you bring in a person who is not emotionally involved with your day-to-day existence—someone who is not a spouse or a close relative—you are bringing much-needed objectivity to your own life. There's really no substitute for objectivity, for the dispassionate, unemotional, clear-eyed perspective that an outsider can bring. So I want to suggest that you find someone whom you think might be a suitable candidate, introduce that person to the ideas behind HDL, and have them read this book. Invite that person to join you on this journey.

What will you do together? You'll keep each other accountable, and thus create a sustainable HDL future for the both of you. Let's say that you've committed to eating only healthy foods. If your HDL accountability partner comes by your home, checks out your kitchen, and finds the shelves groaning under the weight of junk food, then they have the obligation to call you on it.

"What's up with the Twinkies and the ice cream?" your accountability partner says. "I thought you told me you were going to eat healthy!"

Anthony Robbins says that the most successful people are those who convert their "shoulds" to "musts." We can lie to ourselves, dance around the truth, and drop our standards when no one else is looking. But when we know that someone or something is going to keep us accountable, it's a lot easier to turn our shoulds into musts.

Accountability partners can be found in many areas of life. In a religious setting, many church groups create accountability partners to help keep individuals true to their "walk" through life. In this context, accountability partners ensure that the people with whom they are sharing this mission stay true to their spiritual principles. In twelve-step programs, you will also find peer-to-peer accountability in the form of sponsorship. Typically, a newcomer to a twelve-step program either selects or is assigned a sponsor, a mentor figure who keeps that person on the path to achieving and maintaining sobriety or abstinence in the area of focus of that particular twelve-step program. In many cases, if the sponsor and sponsee are together long enough, the roles blur and they end up keeping each other accountable, at which point that hierarchical relationship flattens out into a friendship that's more than a friendship. We're not just talking about fishing buddies or weekend warriors at the community softball game. We're talking about people who understand that their very lives depend upon maintaining the standards that the twelve-step program of which they are members has set.

Therapists, psychologists, and counselors also perform the role of providing accountability, though in those settings, the relationship is generally a one-way street. A couple in marriage counseling recognizes that each week at their session, they will be held accountable for any actions or inactions for which they were responsible. When an outside person is shedding light upon what we do and how we live, we all tend to stand a little straighter, behave a little better, and turn those all-important shoulds into musts.

When we talk about an accountability partner in order to maintain that critically important sense of high HDL, in many ways we're combining the best elements of each of these relationships. There's undeniably a spiritual component to the concept of HDL. When we come from "being" instead of fear, and when we are being our best selves, we are living the way we are intended to live. It is impossible to sustain high HDL while harming others through our actions, whether it's at home or in the workplace. A major component of high HDL is recognizing that we are not alone in the universe; that we have responsibilities to ourselves and to each other; and that spirituality isn't something that takes place only in the context of a meditation ashram, a sanctuary of a church or temple, or a yoga studio. One of my clients once said to me, "Ever since our daughter was born, I've had no time for meditation."

"What are you doing during the time when you used to meditate?" I asked.

"I'm watching the *Goodnight, Moon* video with my baby daughter."

"That's your meditation practice," I told him.

In other words, you can find spirituality in anything you do, and the concept of living spiritually, however you define it, is inseparable from the concept of HDL. So there is absolutely a parallel between the accountability process that you find in the HDL context and the one you find in those who lead fulfilled existences.

We were never meant to go it alone, and we need the help, love, and support of others if we are going to have successful, happy, meaningful lives. Peer-to-peer sharing of vital ideas and, equally important, objective guidance about your life build a successful foundation for maintaining your HDL. Your accountability partner is someone who will listen to you share your thoughts and say, "That's a great idea…that's a great idea…that's a great idea…hey, wait a minute—where'd you come up with *that* one?"

Essentially, you've got accountability and objectivity wrapped up in one special friendship. Your accountability partner is the person who will help you make sure that you are living up to your newfound values of being world-class, of coming from a high HDL. Without that guidance and objectivity, it can be all too easy for us to slip back, one degree at a time, to the old, non-world-class, low HDL way of life. After all, if we've lived and thought one way throughout our entire existences and now we are approaching life from a different direction, it's only natural that the old patterns will remain in place, even after we have read the book and made the commitment to being a high HDL individual.

Two of the areas of life laden with the highest level of emotion are romance and finance—our relationship with our loved one (and by extension, our family), and our relationship with money. These are the areas where low or high HDL is most likely to show up. As I said a moment ago, it is extremely difficult, if not impossible, to remain totally objective about our relationships with loved ones, or about what's going on with our work lives. It's hard for us to set aside our emotions, no matter how cool and calm we think we might be, when we feel that we are being unjustly attacked. In situations like that, the objectivity of an HDL accountability partner makes all the difference. Even when things are working just the way we want them to work, it can still be hard for people to step up and live world-class when they've never done so in the past.

I gave the example earlier of my client who needed a

new car, because he was driving a twenty-year-old vehicle that did not exactly inspire confidence in his patients. This client went through intensely complicated feelings before he was able to pull the trigger and lease the Cadillac STS he really wanted. It's tough to step up! It's especially tough to step up if we don't have the support of a committed friend and HDL accountability partner. We talked earlier about the concept of the committee—that group of voices in your head that gang up on you, tell you that you're not good enough, and otherwise seek to depress you and ruin your day. Sometimes it takes the voice of a committed outsider to help us overrule the committee in our heads. After a while, we groove the process, and it becomes easier to ignore those internal negative voices. The accountability partner is the one who helps us overcome the negativity, or ANTs, and find our own path to greatness.

Finally, there is a therapeutic aspect to the accountability partnership process as well. We want to be very careful when we are serving as accountability partners and not "play God" to the people we are supporting. We are not trained therapists, marriage counselors, or finance planners. But we do know what floats! So when we work with others as accountability partners, we may sometimes find ourselves offering marriage counseling or financial advice. This is undeniably an aspect of accountability, but we have to be very careful not to overstep. Rather, we have to empower our partner to draw his or her own conclusions. The most powerful consultants know how to empower and equip clients with the insights and tools they need, leaving them to understand the costs and payoffs of their actions without judging or invalidating them.

So there you have it—the key to sustaining your new, high HDL is your commitment to sharing what you've learned with others, because that moves you from a 10 to 20 percent retention rate to a 90 to 100 percent retention rate. The relationship between two individuals committed to high HDL is one part empowerment, one part mentorship, and one part cathartic. The total relationship is much greater than the sum of the parts, of course.

Think synergy. Think holistically. Think wholly…and a most holy partnership will come.

Now I want to talk about the power of agreements, which form the fundamental building blocks of your relationships with others.

The beautiful thing about high HDL is that it raises the quality of every aspect of life, from relationships to finance, from health and fitness to career. People with low HDL are in the unfortunate position of, say, making a lot of money but getting divorced ten times, or being in great physical shape but sorely lacking in fiscal or financial fitness. That's why I love the HDL concept so much, because it paves the way to a balanced life where everything in your life is world-class. So the question is how you lock in the benefits that high HDL gives you. And it all comes down to making and keeping agreements.

The problem is that most people in the world don't keep their agreements, either with each other or with themselves. We all know what it takes to eat right and stay in shape, but how many people out there really practice a healthy diet and get enough exercise? We all know that cheating on one's spouse is wrong, but lots of people do it. My wife has said to me, "If you cheat on me, don't come back. It's not a discussion." In other words, her boundaries are really clear. I combine her boundaries with my own moral concepts, and we have an agreement in place. As long as I don't violate that agreement, our marriage can stay strong.

Agreements must be made and kept in all areas of our lives, not just in terms of relationships. It's okay to express to the other person in any situation, business or personal, exactly what the nature of your agreement should be. In fact, it's best when we take the time to establish clear agreements, because then everyone knows how to behave. Your patients need to understand that they must show up on time, pay their bills, and otherwise operate in accordance with the requirements in a relationship that you create. I recommend doing a new patient interview and re-training existing patients on new agreements that you establish so that you can have the practice operate at an optimal level benefiting everyone involved.

Just as you outline your expectations of the patients, your patients have the right to spell out their expectations of you. Clear, written agreements make for the best possible relationships, because you avoid misunderstandings and set appropriate expectations all around. When we work with new clients, they actually have to fill out an eleven-page questionnaire, and each member of their team has to fill out a team survey. The survey spells out key expectations for a successful relationship, and everyone in the office has to review these and agree on them. In addition, the clients pay upfront for the services. That helps us screen out the people who are serious and committed from those who are not ready and might not fully benefit from our services. We then have a session that we describe as, "You interview us and we interview you to see if we will be successful together." Dentists who are going to join our consultancy must meet certain parameters in terms of their desire to make changes, their willingness to take direction, and their financial and emotional stability. If we agree to take them on, we establish our "rules of engagement." Among the requirements: They must stay in communication, keep their agreements, and sleep and eat well! It's impossible to be world-class if you are not getting adequate rest and nutrition. We want them to be in a position to deliver on their promises to their patients, and we believe that can only happen if they deliver on their promises to us.

Being on time is essential. Showing up on time is always the wisest course in any relationship. Our dentists must be on time for their appointments with us. They must fulfill on and deliver on all the things they have agreed to by a certain time. If they send us their practice evaluation and team surveys on time, that signals us as to whether they will be staying punctual throughout our engagement.

You might ask why we are such sticklers for punctuality. To put it simply, how happy are you when your people— your team members, boyfriend, girlfriend, spouse, partner, or colleagues—are consistently late? It's said that when we steal time from another human being, we have created a debt that we can never pay back. You can always pay back

$15, but how do we repay the fifteen minutes that we kept someone else waiting? Lateness, to put it simply, is a sign of disrespect, and people will only tolerate being disrespected for so long before they move on. A successful relationship—a world-class relationship—must be founded on strict adherence to time, because without that, the relationship is not likely to flourish.

You have every right to demand of yourself and those around you that they adhere to the agreements you and they co-create. What's interesting is that it takes a lot of time to clean up the messes in our own lives that we discussed in previous chapters. It takes time to address the leaks in our integrity bucket, to learn to keep our word to ourselves and others, and to identify and live by the moral standards that become guideposts instead of mere wishes. For most people who go through the HDL process, the idea of hanging around in a relationship where agreements are not honored becomes very undesirable. They find that they want to put structures in place in the relationships that survive their move to high HDL, so as to avoid going through the roller coaster all over again. Part of having high HDL is reassessing your relationships on an ongoing basis.

In my business, we review each of our clients annually to make sure that the fit still exists. I understand it's a very different way to look at business, compared with the usual approach of "taking anybody with a credit card and pulse." We do this not because life's too short to work with undesirable people, but because life's too long to have to spend our time creating messes, cleaning them up, and starting all over again.

We've talked mostly about how agreements apply in the work setting. I'd like to briefly discuss how they also apply in relationships by sharing with you a technique my wife and I use. Every year, we sit down and have an end-of-the-year meeting in which we look at our lives and clean up the stuff that's not working. This annual meeting usually takes place "offsite" in a nice spot. On the last day of the year, my wife and I take ourselves one year into the future and look back on how the forthcoming year went. That provides the structure of the conversation. We talk about where we traveled, what we needed, and what had to happen. That way, we're constantly coming from the future instead of the present or the past. This is a very effective technique, and you don't have to wait for New Year's Eve to apply it—you can try it right now, with your team *and* with your significant other.

My wife and I also have regular meetings on a quarterly and a weekly basis to handle things as they arise. In these meetings, we focus on the two sides of our relationship—the intimate, emotional, love side, and then also the business aspects. You most likely marry for love (I hope so, anyway!), but when you commit, you get more than a marriage partner. You get a business partner, because running a home and family is like running a business. You've got vendors, cash flow, tax responsibilities, shopping, cooking, cleaning—the whole nine yards. If you don't have good agreements in place, somebody's going to be unhappy. And as the expression goes, if Mama's unhappy, ain't nobody happy. Since you're managing relationships, friendships, money, and a million and one other things, it's important to keep measuring to ensure that your agreements are being observed.

I put so much emphasis on the concept of agreements because by and large, the world simply doesn't run on agreements. Agreements are not even on most people's radar. But when we put a structure around things and understand that agreements really have a profound effect on everything, life becomes so much easier. Living life without agreements is like trying to drive a car without oil. You're not going to get very far!

What makes agreements so powerful is that they enable you to create a basis for a relationship working on a world-class level, whether it's a personal or a business relationship. That way, when it's not working, you can immediately look back to your agreements to find out where the breakdown has occurred. Once you put in agreements, the world has to dance to your tune. Of course, if you don't keep your agreements, you can't expect others to keep theirs. You can't expect your patients to pay you on time if you are always late yourself. Be accountable. Set the precedent. If patients don't keep their agreements, it's because you have allowed that to happen—you've created a standard of "not keeping agreements" in your environment. That's the act of a low HDL person, which doesn't describe you anymore.

Are agreements the key to instant bliss? Of course not. Once you start putting agreements in place, you'll see push-back. You'll see people looking at you and saying, "Who is this person? He's never operated by agreements before! Why is he expecting me to operate by an agreement now?" You simply have to accept the fact that the world generally does not operate by agreements, and then start educating and enrolling those in your environment to accept the idea that this is how life will be from this moment on.

Once you do this, you'll likely notice the people whom you attract going forward are much more apt to operate by agreements. Everybody likes to criticize lawyers, but one thing lawyers do very well is that they operate on a basis of facts—they cut away all the stories and emotion behind things and focus on what actually happened. If there is a written contract that says you must do XYZ, either you did XYZ or you did not. That's the starting point for figuring things out. So when you have agreements in place, it doesn't mean you're turning into Perry Mason. It just means that you're able to handle things on a more mature level, both at work and at home.

It's best to find ways to "automate" your agreements so that you don't find yourself in the position of watching your standards slowly slip away. A client of mine got himself into a rut and didn't know how to get out because it had taken him so long to get there. One of his team members showed up five minutes late for work one day. The following week, she showed up ten minutes late each day. The weeks after, she started showing up fifteen and twenty minutes late. Then, when he hired a new team member (because his practice was growing), the new team member got the idea that it was acceptable to show up late. As a result, the practice consistently ran behind schedule, things were done in a hurried fashion in the mornings, and the dentist wound up compensating for his team members' lateness by doing their morning jobs. He was sick of it, but he was stuck. He had set the precedent by failing to address the issue immediately. He had been in the situation of having his standards slip away, not all at once, but drop by drop. That's how it happens for all of us—if we don't adhere to our standards, and if we don't automate the standards in our lives, then it's all too easy for us to have those standards slip.

What does it mean to automate your standards? It means bringing in other people who are going to help you keep your agreements. Now we've come back to the concept of having accountability partners. If eating properly is important to you, then you want to see a nutritionist on a monthly or quarterly basis so that you can check in and make sure that you are eating in accordance with your new, higher standards. If a healthy body is important to you, then you want to work out with a personal trainer. If maintaining high standards in your financial life is important, then you want to have regular, ongoing meetings with your financial planner or accountant, not just ad hoc sessions that arise because of a sudden financial crisis or an unexpected tax bill. To the extent that you have regular meetings with people who are able to hold you to the standards you have created for yourself, it will be that much easier for you to maintain your world-class status.

Incidentally, every time you spend money on a worthy cause (like yourself!)—and I'm talking about hiring a consultant or working with a financial planner or some other worthwhile investment—you are enriching those people who are providing you with the services you need. Your outflow of cash to them creates a greater sense of money flowing back to you. It's not just the idea of spending money to make money—it's the idea of investing money in yourself in order to create a sense of flow, which means that others will be spending money to be with you. If you're coming from a meaningful purpose, then by contributing to yourself, you're contributing to others…and still others will contribute back to you.

This is a good moment to stop and ask why people spend money. In an advertising- and consumer-driven culture like ours, people typically spend out of fear. The news media traffics in fear on a minute-by-minute basis. We consume news—and we buy TVs, radios, and computers from which we learn the news—because we've been motivated to do so through fear tactics. By contrast, I'm talking here about spending not out of fear but out of love—love for ourselves, love for others, love for the world. What starts your day? An alarm clock and a cold shower of bad news? Or something inspirational and motivational?

If you chose the first answer, it's time to make a change. Sustaining your high HDL means living a life of passion, enthusiasm, and excitement. In order to do that, you need someone to cheer you on. It's next to impossible to stay on track if you look out into the stands and don't see a single fan in your corner!

Now's the time to find that accountability partner, someone who can bring an objectivity to your life and who will be by your side as you work to sustain your high HDL. In return, you have to be willing to do the same for them. The two of you must work together to keep your agreements, to automate them, and to continue to invest in yourself for a worthy cause. Because the most worthy cause in the world…is simply you.

HDL Highlights

- It's not enough to win—you have to know, in your heart, that you've won.

- At one time or another, most of us have been unwilling to recognize that we deserved the fruits of victory, and unable to experience the sweetness of life, despite the outward trappings we may possess.

- It's not just about creating a high HDL—it's about creating a sustainable HDL.

- A major component of high HDL is recognizing that we are not alone in the universe; that we have responsibilities to ourselves and to each other; and that spirituality isn't something that takes place only in the context of a meditation ashram, a sanctuary of a church or temple, or a yoga studio.

- Your accountability partner is the person who will help you make sure that you are living up to your newfound values of being world-class and coming from a high HDL.

- When we put a structure around things and understand that agreements really have a profound effect on everything, life becomes so much easier.

- You and your accountability partner must work together to add structure to your life; to keep and automate your agreements; and to learn how to invest in yourself for a worthy cause. Because the most worthy cause in the world...is simply you.

■ Chapter 10 Exercise / **Keeping on Track**

1. Find an "accountability partner" for yourself and meet regularly—weekly is best. Educate them about what standards you wish to set for your career, health, relationships, spirituality, personal energy, and environment. Set specific, measurable outcomes so that your partner can hold you accountable for the actions you take that either attract or push away those goals.

2. Tell your accountability partner: "My ideal career looks like…", "My ideal income looks like…", "My ideal body looks like…", and so on. Once you've put words to your goals and actually spoken them aloud to someone else, you're far more likely to achieve them.

3. Keep your agreements with your accountability partner. These are the most important meetings you'll ever have!

4. Sign up for the Morning Huddle Motivator at **www.garykadi.com**.

Nine Qualities of a High HDL Individual

A MAN SAW A COUPLE dancing gracefully in an old black-and-white movie. He thought, wouldn't it be nice if I could dance like that? So he signed up for lessons. At first, he felt awkward, and he feared that he would be the worst dancer in the class. Then it dawned on him that the room was full of people who had never danced before in their lives, or at least who didn't dance particularly well. After all, the class was called "Ballroom Dancing for Beginners." So he realized that he would probably be in the middle of the pack, and he forgot his fears and paid attention to the teacher.

"We're going to do the fox trot," she said. "The steps are like this." She demonstrated the basic fox trot steps, and the line of twenty newcomers to ballroom dance shuffled along with her, awkwardly at first, and then with increasing confidence. She paired the dancers, showed them how to hold their partners' hands, and put the music on.

The man gave his partner a nervous smile and tried to remember the instructor's advice to keep his eyes off his feet. He couldn't help it—he wanted to make sure his feet were going where they were supposed to go. Although he had never danced before, he was agile, and within a few moments, he had reached the next level: he was hearing the music and thinking about his feet, but he wasn't looking at them. Then he reached the next level, the place where his feet were moving him, instead of him directing his feet where to go. Then he and his partner reached the next level, where the music was moving both of them. And then they reached the next level after that, where they weren't just dancing. Dancing became them.

Just like our friend in the ballroom dancing class, you are the dance. You no longer have your attention on yourself. You are just in the present moment, enjoying what's happening around you. You are aware—aware when life is working, when your practice is thriving, and when it is not. You are a high HDL individual, and while it might have seemed awkward at first, back when you feared that you would never "get it," you have. Just as the dancer embodies the music, it flows through you now, and you don't have to force anything. It's not just that you have high HDL. You *are* high HDL. And everything and everyone in your office and your home reflect it.

In this chapter, I want to talk about the nine characteristics of the high HDL individual. At this point, you already possess these characteristics. You don't think about them consciously anymore. But you do embody them, each and every one. And as such, I'd like to share with you all you have become.

The first characteristic of a high HDL individual is certainty. A person with certainty is free from doubt. Most of us live our lives trapped in doubt. If our lives had a theme song, it would be something like "Should I Stay Or Should I Go?" The high HDL individual, on the other hand, lives, acts, and decides from a position of certainty—not a certainty that she will always make the right choice, but certainty that the choice she makes is the best possible one. The best possible choice is the one that reflects her world-class nature, demonstrating to herself and others that she deserves the best because she gives her best, does her best, and is being her best at all times.

One of my clients had a top-notch dental hygienist on her team who initially balked at the idea of pointing out problem areas to patients. Her attitude was that her job was to clean teeth and nothing more. In the approach I teach through *Million Dollar Dentistry*, however, dental hygienists become part of the diagnosis and treatment process by identifying potential problems and putting them up on a video screen to show the doctor and the patient.

"I'm not in sales," she told me. "I'm a healthcare provider."

I suggested to the hygienist that educating patients about their dental health needs was in fact an important part of being a healthcare provider. Nonetheless, she still took on the responsibility with intense frustration and upset.

After the first day, she called and told me, "I've given this thing 110 percent."

"In that case," I replied, "you've given it 10 percent more than you needed to."

That's because a world-class, high HDL individual gives 100 percent...but nothing more. We don't have to "bend over backwards" or stand on our tippy-toes anymore. We're not dancing as fast as we can. Instead, we're moving gracefully, giving our best, and knowing that our best—our 100 percent—is more than good enough. We know that our best will get the job done the right way, even if it's a job that we might not prefer to do. That's certainty.

After the second day, the dental hygienist called me again…and apologized. "It was just new, and a little scary," she said. "I wasn't sure if patients would get mad at me if I told them I saw something that needed attention, because I've never done that before. It turned out they were really grateful.

"They weren't necessarily happy that they needed dental work done," she added, "but I didn't realize how much they trusted me. I really made a difference for my patients the last two days, because otherwise the issues might never have been brought to their attention in a way where they could really hear it."

It's not world-class to sit there and wonder what's going to happen *if*. High HDL people don't live in a world of doubt, of what if, what if, what if. Instead, they live in a world of what is, what is, what is. If they don't know what is, they don't hesitate to ask. This hygienist demonstrated her world-class nature and her high HDL, all because she took a chance on a new approach to her work, gave it all she had, and saw quickly that her efforts brought positive results for the individuals under her care.

The second characteristic of a high HDL individual is compassion. To be compassionate literally means to feel with others. A compassionate person understands what others are feeling, and cares about what they have to say.

This quality is encapsulated in the Hindu phrase, *namaste*. If you've ever taken a yoga class, chances are that the instructor ended the class by offering a small bow to the students, who bowed back and uttered the word namaste. Namaste isn't simply Hindi for, "Thank you for a great class." It actually means, "The divinity in me salutes the divinity in you." A high HDL person consistently recognizes the divinity in others and sees them not as job titles, but as people—real, live human beings with responsibilities and families and aspirations who happen to be holding a specific job at a specific time. By acknowledging the humanity in others, you actually bring out the best in others. The divinity in each of us is waiting to be saluted by the divinity in you.

When you demonstrate compassion, when you acknowledge the divinity of every human being with whom you come in contact, when you can treat the person who serves you coffee with the same fundamental human respect that you would treat Gordon Christiansen or Joe Blaes...then you are truly living a life of compassion. Remember that expression about being kind to the little people on your way up? The high HDL individual recognizes that there is no such thing as a little person, a lesser-than assistant, or a floater (a person who has no real job description, but serves as a utility). All people are worthy; all people are perfect; all people have a divinity within. Understanding that basic fact of existence is the secret to being a compassionate human being.

The third quality of the high HDL individual is complete gratitude. It's so easy to complain about life, often because our expectations of life are so high that there's always something to complain about. In fact, we love to complain so much that it's practically an Olympic sport for many of us. Some of us are never happy unless we find something to complain about!

When we complain, we think we are demonstrating our superiority to the people or organization that created a particular event, product, or service. "Look how smart we are," we're saying when we complain. "We could have done a much better job than they did! Don't they know anything?" We can complain about other people, our spouses or partners, our children, our co-workers, our clients, the economy, our car, the weather…you name it, and there's a way to tear it down and make it smaller. But when you tear other people down, the person who ends up looking the smallest is you.

High HDL people don't need to complain. They don't need to make other people, places, and things smaller in order to make themselves feel bigger. They already feel big because they live their greatness. If something isn't right, they find a quiet way to get the situation handled. They don't go through their lives trashing the lives and hard work of other people. Instead, they demonstrate a high level of gratitude consistent with an awareness of how beautiful life is and how wonderful their own lives are.

One of the benefits of moving from low HDL to high HDL is that you have a basis of comparison. You can remember how you felt before you developed that sense of world-class standards, of how your life looked before you were living in a high HDL way. As a result, when situations arise, not only do you feel gratitude for whatever happens—whether it's the seemingly good or the seemingly bad—but you're grateful for the awareness that you might not have recognized. You can now appreciate the beauty of the situation in a way you never could have done before you developed your high HDL.

For example, let's say you head out to work early in the morning, and you find that your spouse or partner has put a sticky note on the steering wheel of your car saying, "I love you—have a wonderful day at the office!"

The low HDL person says, "It's about time I got a note like that! Do I have to do everything in this relationship?"

The high HDL individual thinks, "I'm so grateful for the love I have in my life. And I'm also grateful for the fact that I now recognize how full of love my life is…and probably always was. I just wasn't paying attention." So the high HDL person actually experiences a "double shot" of gratitude—he's grateful for the situation that is unfolding, and he's grateful for the newfound recognition of a moment that, during his former low Deserve Level days, he would never have recognized in all its grandeur.

The fourth characteristic of being a high HDL person is that of being a visionary. This is closely related to the previous concept of gratitude. We typically say that a visionary is someone who can see into the future, and yet a true visionary is someone who can see the past and the present as well. He recognizes the past and present for what they are—one is a canceled check, and the other is a promissory note.

A visionary is an individual no longer trapped in negative characteristics like anger, fear, manipulation, and self-pity. Instead, she is able to see situations for what they are—opportunities for growth, opportunities for success, or simply opportunities for learning. A visionary in this context is not someone who is necessarily capable of predicting the future. Instead, a visionary is someone whose ability to see and notice has expanded to the point where she sees not just business opportunities, but opportunities for love and service in every moment of her life. Whether it's asking a team member to perform a particular service, asking a patient for a commitment, or learning to dance the fox trot, the high HDL individual lives in a state of heightened awareness. And the more aware we are of life, the more life means to us.

Here's a good example. If you go to a concert at the symphony and you don't know much about the music, it can frankly get a little dull after a few minutes. You find yourself thinking, When is this going to end? How long is this thing supposed to last? Is there an intermission? When am I supposed to applaud? By contrast, an individual who has studied the composers, the compositions, the music history, the music theory, and the styles of the performers—the orchestra, the conductor, the soloists—is going to get much more out of the experience, simply because she has put much more into it. She's not visionary in the sense that she can predict whether there will be an encore. She's visionary in the sense that she is paying attention to everything that is happening. In other words, she is prepared for the moment and therefore enjoys it even more.

It's been said that chance favors the prepared mind. Well, I would add that the prepared mind enjoys life more than the person who stumbles into a good situation. Granted, they both get something out of the concert—or whatever the situation is. But the individual who put the time in to prepare for it will enjoy it even more. I believe that is what it means to be a visionary.

The fifth quality of the high HDL individual is peacefulness. By now, you have reached a level where you actually surrender to the process of being high HDL, of being world-class in your practice and at home. You have taken responsibility for your past and you have caused a new present and a new future for yourself. As a result, you feel extraordinarily peaceful, trusting and knowing that where you are is exactly where you need to be. Even in the eye of the storm, you're as peaceful as if you were sitting on a mountaintop next to a guru or monk. You live peacefully with others and do not intentionally cause upsets at home, at work, or even on the highway. When things are not peaceful in your life, you know how to troubleshoot, and you are fearless about taking action to resolve matters quickly.

The sixth characteristic of the high HDL individual is willingness. You are a willing person—always open, always ready to receive. You do not shut down. You're willing to learn. If you're asked to do something at work out that's out of your comfort zone, you find a way to make it work, because it might just be a better way. A high HDL person says, "Okay, this assignment doesn't exactly dovetail with my expectations about what my job should be, but that doesn't mean I can't make the most of it. There must be a lesson in here for me, because otherwise I would never have been handed this opportunity or responsibility. Let's see what I can make of it."

Most of us operate in a "yes but" mentality, where we

cannot wait to negate the ideas, suggestions, and wisdom of other people. I encourage my clients to take a "yes" attitude and accept every suggestion with grace. Whether you own the practice or work in the office, whether you're a partner or a hygienist, welcome suggestions and opinions of others in an encouraging manner. This doesn't mean that you are obligated to be placed in degrading situations. It does mean that you can have enormous fun trying on different ideas and approaches to see if they fit.

Most of us fall into a rut in our lives, and once we get into a rut, what do we do? Instead of trying to get out, we decorate the rut. We make it all cozy and plan to stay there until retirement. As a high HDL individual, you don't believe in staying trapped in a rut—not for a minute. On the contrary: you're always willing to try something new, whether it's a new road, a new restaurant, or a new approach in the workplace, just to see where it leads. The high HDL individual may not accept every single suggestion, but she's certainly open to seeing what might happen next.

The seventh characteristic of the high HDL individual is what I like to call "undefended." A highly defended individual is one who is incapable of saying or doing the wrong thing. Instead, he scatters blame like rain. This individual doesn't recognize that when he is pointing a finger at someone, three fingers are pointing right back at him.

One characteristic that most of us cannot stand in other people, and yet somehow tolerate in ourselves, is self-righteousness. It all comes back to that compulsive desire to build ourselves up by tearing others down, to making ourselves right—literally, to be *self-righteous*—by making others wrong. The problem is that the characteristics of self-righteousness and being highly defended have a very short shelf life. People get sick of individuals like this and don't want to do business with them or stay in romantic relationships with them, because it's just too much work. If you've ever had a boss, a boyfriend or girlfriend, or a parent who was in the business of making you wrong in order to feel right, you know exactly what I'm talking about.

A world-class, high HDL individual doesn't need to make you wrong in order to feel right. Have you ever noticed at the beach that big birds and small birds coexist on the sand, practically ignorant of each other? They're cognizant of others of their particular species and join together or defend territory only with their own kind. But the big birds pay practically no attention to the little birds. They merely swoop down, catch their prey, and otherwise go about their business, without any regard for what the little birds are doing. In other words, the big birds don't feel a need to make the little birds wrong in order for them to feel big. Somehow they already know they *are* big!

Are we going to take a big bird or little bird approach to life? Do we need to make others weak in order to feel strong? If we do, then we still have some work to do in terms of raising our HDL. A person with low HDL driving an old beater of a car who's stuck in traffic is more often than not looking at the late model luxury cars on the freeway and thinking envious thoughts. The high HDL individual stuck in that same traffic jam is more likely than not listening to something motivational, educational, or entertaining over his car's high performance sound system and is paying no attention to the other cars on the road. The high HDL individual is like a big bird at the beach—he may be vaguely aware of the little birds, but they are not consuming his attention or field of vision. He is focused on his own thoughts, his own goals, and his own dreams, as well as the thoughts, goals, and dreams of those close to him. The high HDL individual is not self-righteous on the one hand or self-consumed on the other. If he's thinking about other people, he's only thinking about them in the context of, "How can I serve them better?"

The eighth characteristic of the high HDL individual is that they are fun. High HDL people love fun. They love to try new things, experiment, travel, challenge themselves, set fitness goals, go to the theater, learn new things, jump out of a plane to go skydiving, or otherwise live their lives to the fullest. There's an old expression that goes, "If you want something done, give it to a busy person." That's because individuals whose lives are full tend to be far more efficient than people with not that much going on. They have to be efficient in order to pack into their lives all of the varied activities, entertainment, and challenges they wish to enjoy along with their workloads. If you have a great idea, you're better off calling a high HDL person than a low HDL person. An individual who is low HDL is going to pooh-pooh the idea, or tell you that it's not worth doing, or that there's no time, no point, no enjoyment, no juice in it. By contrast, the high HDL individual loves fun so much that she's likely to say, "Let's go for it! I never thought of doing that, but that sounds like it could be a good time. When do we leave?"

As a high HDL individual, you've given up the sense that life is a form of punishment, and that if you aren't hurting or suffering, you aren't doing it the right way. As a high HDL dental professional, you recognize that the fun and the juice of life come to those who take the time to try new things. You bring this attitude into the office and transmit this higher level of positive energy to every patient and coworker with whom you come into contact.

High HDL individuals do not suffer from a Calvinistic sense of guilt or need for self-flagellation—they just go out there and have a good time. They recognize that the yin of work requires the yang of rest and play, and they bring a sense of playfulness to every aspect of their work. They love what they do, and they often enjoy it so much that the idea of retirement is anathema to them. They feel the same way the great architect Philip Johnson did on his eighty-second birthday, when his friends asked him why he didn't retire. "When I can keep on making great buildings," he told them, "why would I just want to make sandcastles at the beach?"

The final characteristic of the high HDL individual is openness. Openness finds expression in many different contexts. As a person with high HDL, you are open to new ideas. You are open to the perspectives and points of view of everyone—your patients, colleagues, competing dentists, partners, and friends. You are open to what others have to say, because close-mindedness gets us deeply into trouble.

High HDL individuals don't necessarily believe that they know best, or that they know the most about any particular topic. They are always willing to learn from others, even people who might be younger or less experienced. They ask questions. They're willing to learn and grow. They're willing to see what you have to say, because of that namaste concept—they recognize that you possess not just your own wisdom and experience, but also an inner sacredness. People with high HDL always assume that they just might be hearing the voice of the Divine through the voice of another human being.

So there you have it—the nine characteristics of the high HDL individual:

- Certainty
- Compassion
- Gratitude
- Visionary
- Peacefulness
- Willingness
- Undefended
- Fun-loving
- Openness

I strongly believe that each of us is born with all of these characteristics, and the process of raising our HDL is simply about getting us back in touch with the characteristics we already possess. Some of us have a higher potential for success than others, but it doesn't mean that we always follow through with the potential we have been given. For every Kobe Bryant or LeBron James, there are dozens of equally talented individuals who never got their game beyond the playground level. Certain people do have enormous genetic or family advantages conferred upon them. We don't all possess the focus of a Tiger Woods or the particular body makeup of a Michael Phelps—short legs and a long torso, mimicking a fish. But what these individuals really possess, and what they have in common with one another, is a burning desire to be the absolute best at what they can be in life. That's equally true of every high HDL individual, even those who have never swung a golf club or swum a lap in a pool.

Earlier we talked about how the Reverend Jesse Jackson, in his rousing speech at the 1988 Democratic National Convention, spoke of the "me that makes me me"—the specific internal makeup of character, desire, and will, combined with life experience and education, that made him unique. Each of us has a "me that makes me me," and we each possess all of the characteristics of the high HDL individual. It's just a question of whether we are willing to take the time to develop them, and, once we've developed them, to allow them to shine through.

The beautiful thing about the process of raising your HDL is that all of these characteristics increase in dimension automatically. It's not as though we have to spend a certain amount of time becoming more fun, or more open-minded, or less self-righteous. As long as we are willing to grow our HDL, these traits grow within us automatically. And when they do, we are able to create great results not just for ourselves but for others. When you raise your HDL, it is simply impossible not to become more compassionate, grateful, peaceful, and visionary. It's all but impossible to remain in worry and fear, the qualities of the non-high

HDL person. Once you become certain, once your mind quiets, you become present to what needs to be done in your life, and you are able to do it without effort.

This happened for me in my work as a consultant. My own personal breakthrough came in terms of my ability to trust myself and be certain about my ability. As I did so, I was able to demonstrate that trust and confidence to others, and that brought me to the point where I was able to create this concept of high HDL and share it with other dentists.

The alternative is stark. We can stay in a low HDL state, work hard, not trust ourselves or others, and keep on using up time and energy until these vital resources are depleted. We can live without enthusiasm. We can live without excitement. We can live without peace or gratitude, and we can spend our whole day making people wrong. But why would we? Where's the fun, the excitement, the juice in that?

One of my clients is a dentist who used to work around the clock. He spent his time staying at the office late, reading up on all the newest scientific and technological developments, and constantly interfering with the satellite office that his partner ran by trying to control all operations remotely. He wasn't around for his family because he didn't trust himself to produce income unless he was working endless hours of every day. Whatever the problem was, he believed that working harder was the answer. He actually moved away from his immediate family to be closer to his business partner, trying to control that team because he did not trust himself.

Once he developed a sense of certainty and began to trust himself, he began to trust his team as well. He became understanding when people made mistakes. He stopped being a perfectionist. He gave people room to explore and grow. His attrition rate—his rate of losing employees—dropped dramatically. His partner and team members began to like working with him, because now he was able to create a place where people respected themselves at work. He had become a visionary. He actually went from $1.2 million to $2 million in his practice in a matter of two years. He had more fun, and more money to spend on having fun. He put in structures and controls that did not require his presence 24/7, because he felt that he deserved to be with his family.

His life is now founded on trust—he trusts himself and his team. He has control without having to be there. He was able to create certainty for his family in terms of income and his own personal availability, and one thing a wife wants from a husband is certainty—both emotionally and financially. My client's wife wanted to know that the money would be there…and she wanted to know that *he* would be there! As a result, not only did his practice and his income improve, but so did his marriage and his relationship with his family.

I want you to do something right now. Get an index card, and write out the nine characteristics of the high HDL individual—certainty, compassion, gratitude, being a visionary, peacefulness, willingness, undefended, fun-loving, and openness. Keep that card in your wallet or purse, at your bedside, on the mirror in your bathroom, or on your desk at work. You can even put it on the dashboard of your car! (Don't worry: it doesn't count as clutter.) The point is, you want it to remind you of who you have become, because high HDL is not simply about making more money or working fewer hours or running a practice or a division more efficiently. It's about becoming a human being in the broadest sense of the word. It's about maximizing on all of your skills, abilities, gifts, and, most of all, your enjoyment of life.

Are you going to feel great about your life? Of course you will. And why not? Everything you've ever wanted is waiting for you—your biggest dreams, your wildest wishes, and the fullest picture of what your life can be. So what are you waiting for? It's yours for the taking!

HDL Highlights

- You now embody the nine characteristics of the high HDL individual.

- The first characteristic of a high HDL individual is **certainty**. A person with certainty is free from doubt.

- The second characteristic of a high HDL individual is **compassion**. To be compassionate literally means to feel with others. Being compassionate means that you understand what others are feeling and care about what they have to say.

- The third quality of the high HDL individual is complete **gratitude**. Instead of complaining or cutting others down, you feel supremely thankful for all the things in your life.

- The fourth characteristic of being a high HDL person is that of being a **visionary**. A visionary is an individual no longer trapped in negative characteristics like anger, fear, manipulation, and self-pity. As a visionary, you are prepared for the future.

- The fifth quality of the high HDL individual is **peacefulness**. By now, you have reached a level where you actually surrender to the process of being high HDL, of being world-class.

- The sixth characteristic of the high HDL individual is **willingness**. You are a willing person, always open, always ready to receive.

- The seventh characteristic of the high HDL individual is what I like to call "**undefended**." Instead of being self-righteous, you don't have to make other people wrong in order to feel right.

- The eighth characteristic of the high HDL individual is that they are **fun**. You've given up the sense that life is a form of punishment, and that if you aren't hurting or suffering, you aren't doing it the right way. On the contrary: you recognize that the fun and the juice of life come to those who take the time to try new things.

- The ninth characteristic of the high HDL individual is **openness**. You are willing to grow, listen, and receive. And remember... every time you interact with another human being, you just might be hearing the voice of the Divine.

■ Chapter 11 Exercise / **The Nine Qualities of a High HDL Individual**

Write a few sentences on each of these aspects of being, and post the list in a high-traffic area in your office and in your home. In other words, make yourself accountable to others to live up to your own standards. Have your team members do the same exercise individually and as a team, and post those as well.

1. Certainty_____

_____

_____

2. Compassion_____

_____

_____

3. Gratitude_____

_____

_____

4. Visionary_____

_____

_____

5. Peacefulness_____

_____

_____

6. Willingness_____

_____

_____

7. Undefended_____

_____

_____

8. Fun-loving_____

_____

_____

9. Openness_____

_____

_____

Chapter 12

Pass It On!

S O NOW YOU'RE WORLD-CLASS! Everything about
you, from the shoes you wear to the way you comb
your hair, says that you are a force to be reckoned with,
a person who "gets it." You're the attractive kind of individual
with whom people would like to pursue business
and personal relationships. Congratulations! You've
accomplished something incredibly wonderful—you've
gotten in touch with what Pat Riley calls the "winner within."
You've acknowledged and have become comfortable living
your greatness. You are maximizing in every aspect of your
life, from romance to finance, from work to leisure time
activities. You have it all...because you are comfortable
being the kind of person who can have it all and enjoy it.

It's amazing how many people believe in negative mantras
like, "You can never get all your ducks in a row," or,
"Three steps backward, one step forward." One of the many
beautiful things about having a high HDL is that you realize
that you absolutely can have all your ducks lined up in

a row. You don't have to be the kind of person who is succeeding in one area and failing miserably in others. You've moved from a "this or that" mentality, which says that you can only have success in one domain of life at the expense of success in others, to a "this *and* that" mentality, which states that success is possible in all areas at the same time. That's pretty sweet!

I truly believe this is the way we were intended to live. Take a look at the world around you—not the steel and glass, concrete and cement world that man creates, but a scene in nature where man's interference is undetectable. It is the essence of everything in nature to grow, to live abundantly, and to grow and live abundantly with ease. Life was never meant to be a struggle. Perhaps in the Cro-Magnon era, but the last time we checked, human beings have evolved somewhat. Yes, there is still strife, enmity, poverty, and war in the world. Just imagine if all the world's leaders had a high HDL and did not need to make others in their society…or their neighbors…or anyone else on the planet wrong. If there were an easy path to creating peace in the Middle East, or removing starvation from Africa, this would be it! Just move the leaders to a high HDL, and stand back and watch what happens. This is what the World Hunger Project is all about—empowering women as key agents of change to work to raise HDL among all.

As interested as I am in sharing the blessings of the high HDL concept with the world, I'm most interested right now in the fact that I've had the opportunity to share it with you. It's your development that I care most about. Even though you and I have likely never met, we're kindred souls. We think the same way—we want the most out of life, and we are not willing to compromise on our dreams and visions, on our integrity, on our agreements, or in our relationships. We desire the best, and we fully grasp on a cellular level that we are entitled to the best. We are playing the biggest game of our lives, and we find incredible joy, excitement, and juice from being on the court instead of watching from the sidelines.

So let's review what we've accomplished in this book. In the first part, Seeing It, we talked about the importance of recognizing that the high HDL concept was the missing piece in your life and in the lives of all the people with whom you interact on a daily basis. Thousands of dentists have attended self-help seminars, gone to therapists, or taken other forms of positive steps in their lives, but they still weren't able to put it all together. Why? Because they lacked the knowledge of the basic concept that you have taken to heart in this book: the idea of HDL.

As we discussed in Part I, distinguishing HDL is often the missing link for dentistry team members, individuals, and couples who have not been maximizing in terms of the quality of their relationships, income, or other measures of success. We also saw that the world is an abundant place and that we are meant to enjoy its marvelous abundance. We talked about how, in order to get where we want to go in life, we have to stop coming from a sense of lack or poverty thinking. Then we examined the ways in which we narcotize ourselves with material things, unfulfilling relationships, or the pursuit of money for its own sake. Whatever substance we've been putting in our I.V.s, it's ultimately not in our best interests. By putting all those ideas together, we were able to see that we were not coming from a place of high HDL.

So then we moved to the second part of the book, Freeing It, in which we began to free ourselves from the grip of a low HDL. We began a clean-up process—we cleaned up our word, our agreements with others, our integrity, our physical spaces like our workspaces, our homes and our cars, and our relationships with other people. We put things on a different plane in order to pave the way for our new, high HDL to sweep in and save the day.

Then, in Part III, we began to be it—we began to live in a high HDL manner. Chances are, if you're like a number of my clients, there was a moment that occurred while you were reading this book when you were suddenly confronted with the fact that you had been handling a particular situation in a low HDL manner. We worked the process step-by-step, but enlightenment usually comes in a lightning-like burst, when suddenly we realize that there is a different way to live our lives. The bolt hits, and in that flash, we see a new alternative for handling a particular situation, or a new approach for creating and maintaining agreements with ourselves and others. In that lightning-like moment, everything changed. We suddenly realized just how world-class we were. We became in tune with the infinite greatness within us. Once that moment occurs, it is impossible to go back.

Let me hedge that last sweeping remark—it *is* possible for us to lower our standards bit by bit. That's why we discussed in this section the importance of maintaining our agreements, automating them wherever possible, and living up to them constantly, so that we could be our best possible selves and inspire others around us to do likewise. We saw the nine characteristics of the high HDL person, and we committed to being those characteristics on a daily basis in all facets of our lives. We also put in the structures and accountability practices that will maintain and sustain our high HDL.

So now we come to the last suggestion that I would like to share with you. The easiest way to maintain and grow your own HDL is to share this concept with others. Human beings were meant to serve one another, not simply to take from one another. You now have something wonderful to share with those around you. Inspire others through your words and deeds to become high HDL people, but don't hesitate to share with them the specifics of the program you have found in this book. Imagine if everyone in your world came from a place of high HDL in everything they did. What kind of world do you think that would be? A pretty great one, I would think!

So what do you need to do to contribute to the world around you? Share the ideas you've found here. And let me know how your life and the lives of those around you have taken on new meaning, new significance, new success, and new joy. I'll be looking forward to hearing from you, and as you embrace your own world-class nature, namaste—the divinity in me salutes the divinity in you. I wish you every great success.

HDL Highlights

- It is the essence of everything in nature to grow, to live abundantly, and to grow and live abundantly with ease. Life was never meant to be a struggle.

- As individuals with a high HDL, we want the most out of life, and we are not willing to compromise on our dreams and visions, on our integrity, on our agreements, or in our relationships to get it.

- We desire the best, and we fully grasp on a cellular level that we are entitled to the best.

- We are playing the biggest game of our lives now, and we find incredible joy, excitement, and juice from being on the court instead of watching from the sidelines.

- Enlightenment usually comes in a lightning-like burst, when suddenly we realize that there is a different way to live our lives. The bolt hits, and in that flash, we see a new alternative to handling a particular situation, or a new approach for creating and maintaining agreements with ourselves and others.

- The easiest way to maintain and grow your own HDL is to share this concept with others.

- Inspire others through your words and deeds to become high HDL people, but don't hesitate to share with them the specifics of the program you have found in this book.

■ Chapter 12 Exercise / **Pass It On!**

Share wins with others from living the nine characteristics of a high HDL individual. Don't keep the good news to yourself. Introduce the concept of HDL to your study club, morning huddles, and team meetings. Help others find accountability partners.

Spread the wealth. Most of all, enjoy life and have fun!

Send your HDL success stories to me, Gary, at **successes@garykadi.com.**

Continuing the Conversation

If you're interested in giving your HDL a boost when you wake up every morning, go to **www.garykadi. com** and sign up for an automated process that sends you a motivational, positive thought for the day. Feed your mind warmth, motivation, and inspiration…or feed your mind fear. The choice is always yours.

In addition to the free, daily motivational message that we share with our clients and friends, we also provide a higher, more personalized level of accountability. The model we base this on is that of distance athlete coaches like Chris Carmichael, who worked with Lance Armstrong for many years. Just as you can get a training program for triathlons or multi-day bicycle races online with trainers like Carmichael, we would be happy to tailor a specific program to your needs in order to help you raise your HDL.

At **www.garykadi.com**, you'll discover more inform- ation about our services. You can join our community, take part in our Leading Dentists of the World bulletin board, and find accountability partners, coaches, and mastermind groups. We also offer workshops on various topics related to high HDL, and by becoming a part of the community, you can take advantage of those as well. I look forward to seeing you there!